Seamless Connections

Refocusing Your Organization to Create a Successful Continuum of Care

Connie J. Evashwick, ScD

Foreword by Philip A. Newbold

American Hospital Publishing, Inc.
An American Hospital Association Company
Chicago

This publication is designed to provide accurate and authoritative information in regard to the subject matter covered. It is sold with the understanding that neither the authors nor the publisher is engaged in rendering legal, accounting, or other professional service. If legal advice or other expert assistance is required, the services of a competent professional person should be sought.

The views expressed in this publication are strictly those of the authors and do not necessarily represent official positions of the American Hospital Association.

Library of Congress Cataloging-in-Publication Data

Evashwick, Connie.
    Seamless connections : refocusing your organization to create a successful continuum of care / Connie J. Evashwick.
        p.   cm.
    Includes bibliographical references.
    ISBN 1-55648-183-7
    1. Hospitals—Case management services. 2. Continuum of care.
I. Title.
    [DNLM: 1. Continuity of Patient Care—organization & administration. 2. Primary Health Care—organization & administration. 3. Patient Care Team—organization & administration.   W 84.6 E925s 1997]
    RA975.5.C36E933 1997
    362.1'1'068—dc21
    DNLM/DLC
    for Library of Congress   96-29703
                                                                        CIP

Catalog no. 067105

Printed in the USA

©1997 by American Hospital Publishing, Inc., an American Hospital Association company.

АНА is a service mark of the American Hospital Association used under license by American Hospital Publishing, Inc.

Cover design by Jeanne Calabrese Design

Discounts on bulk quantities of books published by American Hospital Publishing, Inc. (AHPI), are available to professional associations, special marketers, educators, trainers, and others. For details and discount information contact:
American Hospital Publishing, Inc.
Books Division
737 North Michigan Avenue
Chicago, Illinois 60611-2615   FAX 312/951-8491

To the friends and colleagues with whom I've worked
over the past 18 years who have dedicated their
professional energies to building continuums of care.
May our efforts prove worthwhile!

Contents

About the Author

Connie J. Evashwick, ScD, FACHE, is the endowed chair and director of the Center for Health Care Innovation at California State University in Long Beach. Dr. Evashwick holds a bachelor's and a master's degree from Stanford University and a master's and doctoral degree from the Harvard School of Public Health. She is a Fellow of the American College of Healthcare Executives and a licensed nursing home administrator. Since 1983, Dr. Evashwick has worked with more than 35 hospitals, health systems, and nursing homes to develop strategic plans for a continuum of care. Her experience in direct operations includes managing a hospital geriatrics department, developing innovative home care programs, and directing corporate-level units on aging and long-term care. Previous positions include: vice president of long-term care for the Eastern Mercy Health System, director of the Office on Aging and Long-Term Care of the American Hospital Association, and vice president of long-term care for the Lutheran Hospital Society of Southern California. Dr. Evashwick has authored over 70 publications. She coedited the 1987 book, *Managing the Continuum of Care* and edited the 1995 textbook, *The Continuum of Long-Term Care: An Integrated Systems Approach.*

Foreword

The day is not too far away when you will rush in a few minutes late to your child's soccer game. As you push through the crowd to get to your seat, excusing yourself along the way for blocking the view of several of your parent companions, you will likely mutter something to the effect of "I'm sorry I'm late, I just got off work." Someone beside you will say, "That's alright," and may even ask where you work. "At Memorial," you will respond. Your answer will not have told them much; they still will have no idea where you work or what you do. After all, you could be working in any number of places—a school system, helping kids and parents make healthier choices and adopt healthier behaviors and lifestyles; a congregation, helping members become more self-sufficient in terms of their own health or teaching them to use the existing health care system more appropriately and productively; the neighborhood, helping to organize outreach services, bring health care closer to where people live, and improve individual family structures; a work site, teaching people how to adopt healthier behaviors on the job or reengineering their jobs to improve health and reduce injury; a recreation or senior center, teaching people to practice prevention and improving participation in screenings and early detection services so as to minimize the amount of illness and injury they experience; an ambulatory or urgent care center or a physician's office, helping people to stay healthier and supplement much of their education with classes on prevention and complementary medicine techniques; or the home, helping people to enjoy the benefits of their home environment and live as independently and productively as possible.

In the future, only about half the people who work at Memorial will work in an inpatient facility or at the bedside. The other half will work outside the traditional walls of the hospital, keeping people healthier, educating them to make healthy choices, and providing an environment in which they can grow mentally, physically, and spiritually throughout their lifetimes. This future scenario is rapidly being implemented in progressive health care systems throughout the country. Increasingly, people want to be more self-sufficient, less dependent on an acute care system, and able to live their lives more productively with existing chronic conditions. Care managers, wellness coaches, and health and lifestyle assistants will be an emerging group of individuals who will help build the connection points between existing acute care, chronic care, long-term care, and ambulatory care settings.

Seamless Connections: Refocusing Your Organization to Create a Successful Continuum of Care does an impressive job of outlining how the new continuum will be planned, organized, and implemented with all of today's emphasis on deal making and acquisitions. The real challenge will be in making organizations actually implement meaningful changes. The book carefully lays out the major operational issues that arise in implementing the continuum and describes the range of practical steps and actions that should be taken to achieve future success. This book is about how to make the important connections in building a continuum. It is about the interfaces between the various health care services that need practical solutions and innovative approaches. Whether you are in a leadership capacity with a single hospital, a multi-entity health system, a home health agency, or some other health care entity, this book will offer practical steps and implementation strategies for tomorrow's organizations.

Leaders who pay close attention to the concrete examples and case studies provided in this book will find real value added by the practical actions suggested. Quality of care will be greatly improved, patients will be more satisfied with their care, and operating efficiencies will be realized with these well-thought-out strategies. I strongly recommend that health care leaders pay close attention to the advice and lessons learned as they create and implement a seamless continuum of care. Our community organizations and those whom we serve will be better served as a result of the successful implementation of these tools for change.

Philip A. Newbold

President and Chief Executive Officer
Memorial Health System, Inc.
South Bend, Indiana
1996

Preface

During the past 15 years, many health care organizations have developed strategic plans and initiated actions designed to create a continuum of care. Although one would think that by now all organizations functioned as a seamless and complete continuum, the reality is that, to date, few have succeeded in doing so. However, as consumers become more sophisticated in their demands for comprehensiveness and continuity of care, and as managed care offers incentives for providers to assume broad responsibility for keeping members healthy, creating a seamless continuum of care will be more important than ever for those organizations striving to succeed in the marketplace of the 21st century.

The purpose of this book is to alert senior managers to the basic operating issues their organization will encounter as it implements a continuum of care. By emphasizing the pragmatic aspects of creating a continuum, it attempts to help senior managers anticipate the consequences of their decisions at the department level or the clinical bedside. However, the book's intent is not to present a single, cookie-cutter way to handle each issue but, rather, to raise management awareness of the issues that should be addressed by the organization and to present examples of techniques that other organizations have used to address those issues.

I would like to thank those who willingly shared their creativity in brainstorming ideas and contributed their time by reviewing drafts: Richard Bringewatt, Ellen Browne, David Coile, Craig Duncan, Timmothy Holt, Audrey Kaufman, Charles Kondis, Joan Kwiatkowski, Jeanne Lally, George Mack, Barbara McCandless, Donna Melkonian, Philip Newbold, DeWayne Oberlander, Ed jj Olson, Deborah Paone, Kimberly Smith, Roberta Suber, Rose Marie Tracy, Monika White, Nancy Whitelaw, and Rick Zawadski. My special thanks to Charles Kondis, Jeanne Lally, Cheryl Schraeder, and Paul Shelton for authoring the case studies. Finally, I would like to thank the many health care professionals throughout the nation with whom I have worked during the past 15 years, and who have shared with me their frustrations and triumphs in attempting to create continuums of care.

Introduction

Those who study organizations have articulated theories that help explain the rationale for the continuum of care and why the task of creating one is more daunting than might be expected. According to organizational behavior and systems theories, organizations may be depicted as a three-way alliance of tasks, people, and structure.[1] Inputs enter the organization, are modified by the tasks the people perform operating under the specified structure, and outputs are produced. Surrounding the organization is an environment comprising an array of factors over which the organization may have little control, such as politics, economics, religion, and culture.[2]

The environment surrounding health care delivery in the United States has changed dramatically. Financing for health care has gone from being primarily indemnity insurance and seemingly unlimited government programs to managed care and severely constrained government programs. These changes alone would cause change in organizational structure and tasks. But there are other factors at work. The health care organization that once was able to function more or less in peaceful isolation now is irrevocably subject to external penetration and inextricably linked in a web of interdependencies: community coalitions, parent corporations, affiliated companies. The information technology explosion has brought interaction of all types and both benefits and challenges for the organization. Moreover, the inputs and the desired outputs have changed. Patients entering the health care system are more likely to be enrollee members who are either healthy or suffering from long-term, chronic illness than people experiencing acute illness. Similarly, rather than cure from an acute episode of illness, we now expect our health care system to promote wellness and to care for the chronically ill over time. As managed care expands and community–benefit pressures heat up, the unit of output changes from the individual patient to an enrolled population—or even an entire community.

Structuring health care as a continuum and accepting the goal of providing comprehensive, ongoing care for a large number of people whose conditions range from well to chronically ill is a radical change for the health care system. This change requires that the structures, tasks, and people within the organization change. Indeed, creating a continuum of care is really about changing all aspects of an organization to accept this new orientation. Tasks become not those that can be done in isolation but, rather, those that must be done collaboratively with people in other organizations. Traditional structures, such as lines of authority, must be revamped to accommodate positions and tasks that span components both within an organization and across many organizations. People must become comfortable with jobs that did not exist several years ago, with creating new roles, and with resolving turf battles that try to protect old domains.

Thus, the principles of organizational change are fundamental to the creation of a seamless continuum. Participation, education, and ongoing communication are essential to helping board, staff, physicians, and consumers understand and accept new roles and responsibilities, and must be done on an ongoing basis to accommodate the constant evolution of the organization, the changing loyalties of patients, the job moves of staff, and the continuous realliance of organizational affiliations.

Structure of the Book

Seamless Connections: Refocusing Your Organization to Create a Successful Continuum of Care is divided into three parts: definition (chapter 1), operational issues (chapters 2 through 13), and case studies (chapters 14 through 16). Chapter 1, "The Continuum of Care Concept," defines a continuum of care as being more than a collection of independent services and stresses the importance of its integrating mechanisms and ability to guide and track clients over time. Those who would undertake a continuum must understand what they are trying to create and how it differs from the current mode of care. The definition includes health, mental health, and social services spanning all levels of care brought together by four basic integrating mechanisms: structure, clinical coordination, information systems, and financing.

The first of the issues chapters, chapter 2, "Consensus and Commitment," highlights the importance of mission, goals and objectives, and leadership in building support within the organization for the continuum and the changes it will bring. Chapter 3, "Patient/Client Focus," discusses issues pertaining to targeting a patient population. Once in place, the mechanics and processes of a continuum can be applied to multiple target groups and will benefit all constituencies. Chapter 4, "Services of the Continuum," describes the issues involved in identifying the services that will comprise the continuum. The organization need not own or operate all services, but it must give its patients/clients/ enrollees access to a full spectrum of services. Chapter 5, "Structure and Management," presents issues pertaining to the first of the four integrating mechanisms—how to structure the relationships among many services (total single ownership, collaboratives, affiliation agreements) and the management considerations that are affected by structure. Chapter 6, "Human Resources," one aspect of structural integration, deals with the myriad "people" issues that arise in trying to meld services provided by different organizations, with different pay scales, types of personnel, and cultures. Chapters 7, "Case Management," and 8, "Other Types of Care Coordination," describe the second of the four integrating mechanisms—coordinating clinical care. As chapter 7 explains, case management has not only become accepted in the past decade but has proliferated. Chapter 8 describes other approaches to coordinating clinical care, including interdisciplinary teams, single-entry access, and integrated records. Chapter 9, "Information Systems," discusses the third integrating mechanism: the data systems needed to guide and track patients through a comprehensive array of services over time and describes the benefits of, and challenges inherent in, creating an integrated medical record. The fourth integrating mechanism, finance, is covered in chapters 10, "Financing the Continuum," and 11, "Managed Care." Chapter 10 treats operating finance issues such as how to pay for a continuum of services when dollars are allocated according to a fragmented array of payers and their concomitant restrictions. Chapter 11 presents those issues that arise due to managed care, which offers both the potential to aggregate funds and to fragment care further. Chapter 12, "Marketing," focuses on the ultimate aspect of structural integration: getting the word out to professionals and consumers alike, explaining what the continuum is and how it can benefit them. And finally, the last of the issues chapters, chapter 13, "Evaluation," raises some of the yet-unanswered questions about evaluating the continuum.

The chapters in the book's last section describe the experiences of three organizations that are well advanced in the process of successfully implementing a continuum of care—The Carle Clinic Association, in Urbana, Illinois; Mercy Medical, in Daphne, Alabama; and Fairview, in Minneapolis. Finally, chapter 17 concludes the book. Throughout the book many illustrations are used. All are real examples of individual organizations or composites of the actual experiences of several organizations.

Caveats about the Book

In putting together a book on a subject as complex as the continuum of care, many decisions must be made in order to bring focus to a broad subject within a limited space. As you read this book, keep the following in mind.

First, this is not a technical reference. Instead, it provides an overview of what happens throughout all aspects of continuum implementation so that experts in one area might come to understand the operations issues being dealt with by their colleagues in other areas and find ways to work together to address the overall issues of creating a continuum. Also, this book does not pretend to be complete: Many more issues and examples could be delineated in each chapter. Rather, the book is more of a guide to remind senior administrators that operating details ultimately make or break success.

Second, discussion of each operational issue in the book is followed by a set of recommended actions, some of which apply to all organizations and some of which represent choices. Similarly, some are sequential, and others are not. The intent is to give a range of action options that will enable readers to find something applicable to their specific situations without being totally prescriptive. Throughout, the potential actions include recommendations for committees and task forces. As much as we all cringe at the thought of establishing yet another committee, the core principles of the continuum include the notion that services are comprehensive and coordinated. Thus, it is imperative to establish ways for clinicians and administrators to communicate, both for planning/development and on an ongoing basis—and committees are the customary way to do this. Although a designated continuum director should be granted authority to make day-to-day decisions, a single administrator can never bring all the perspectives required for the continuum. In clinical care and in administration, the continuum implies a team approach to care. For some health care and social service professionals, this may be an uncomfortable modus operandi, but a successful future depends on organizations and individuals learning to work together on a daily basis to plan the long-term direction of the health care delivery systems of the 21st century.

Third, in talking about the continuum, finding the most appropriate terminology is tricky. For example, is the user of the service a client, a patient, a customer, a resident, or a consumer? Assuming that the majority of readers are from health care provider organizations and that the majority of users come into the system when they are ill, the term *patient* seemed the likely term of choice. Ideally, of course, the continuum will include both the residential and wellness aspects of a person's life. Once a person identifies with the continuum, whether through enrollment in a health plan or an unexpected visit to an emergency department, it will likely have outreach programs that from then on will actively focus on keeping that person healthy.

Another terminology issue centers on what to call the components of the continuum. These may consist of service divisions of a large multi–health care system, community agencies affiliated in a network, or departments within a single community hospital. Formal relationships may be ownership, affiliation, contractual, or an array of combinations. Because the goal of the continuum is to provide access to the services people need when they need them, a vast spectrum of services is needed, and the organizational forms those services take are likely to vary even within a single continuum. In this book, the term *participating entity* is used to refer to the services, individual providers, payers, and others who are directly involved with a given continuum of care.

Fourth, try as one might, it is difficult to accommodate all perspectives in a single book. The concept of the continuum applies equally well in small communities as in large ones. It applies to affiliations of community-based, primarily social service agencies; to networks of mental health agencies; to community hospitals working with private medical groups; and to large multi–health care systems. The driving force may come from acute or long-term care or residential services, or from government, public, or not-for-profit entities. Although this book is written primarily for administrators of hospitals and health systems, it is hoped that administrators of nursing homes, home health agencies, social service programs, medical groups, and health plans, too, will find information that is relevant and useful, and will not be offended at the focus on the hospital as the driver of the continuum of care. Indeed, many examples exist of excellent continuums being driven by lead organizations other than hospitals. In the end, all types of providers must cooperate if the continuum is to achieve the ultimate goal of seamless access to all potentially needed services.

And finally, many of the suggestions in this book are elementary management techniques. They are hardly earthshaking, nor should they be "organization-shaking." However, they are often overlooked. The underlying approach to creating a continuum is common management sense:

- Define what the continuum will be.
- Delineate goals and objectives.
- Co-opt all the key stakeholders.
- Communicate with all involved, including staff, physicians, board, and consumers.
- Secure or cultivate staff expertise consistent with the requisite tasks.
- Structure authorities and management processes to reflect tasks.
- Reinforce successes.
- Evaluate and modify as needed.

Very simple! The art is in doing it!

References

1. Etzioni, A. *Modern Organizations.* New York City: Prentice-Hall, 1964.

2. Lawrence, P., and Lorsch, J. *Organization and Environment.* Homewood, IL: Irwin, 1969.

Part One

Definition

Chapter 1

The Continuum of Care Concept

A *continuum of care* is a client-oriented system of care composed of both services and integrating mechanisms that guides and tracks clients over time through a comprehensive array of health, mental health, and social services spanning all levels of intensity of care.[1] The components of this definition are intentional.

"Client-oriented" means that the continuum is organized in a way that best meets the needs of users, not providers or payers. Clients want the illusive quality of "seamlessness," which means that they do not want to go through the admissions process seven different times, get separate bills from a dozen different services, or wonder which provider to call when they feel ill. A continuum organized around the needs of a particular target population is likely to be the most effective and efficient way of organizing care.

The "services" of the continuum vary according to the characteristics, needs, and preferences of the client population. Figure 1-1 shows more than 50 different services that may be needed by a person during spells of both illness and wellness. A single entity may not own or operate every service, but it can give its clients access to the services they need when they need them. For simplicity, our model identifies seven major types of services: extended care, acute care, ambulatory care, home care, outreach, wellness, and housing.

Services alone do not make a continuum! "Integrating mechanisms" are the management techniques essential to the smooth, efficient operation of the continuum. The continuum of care model identifies four basic integrating mechanisms: interservice planning and management, care coordination, integrated information systems, and integrated financing. Figure 1-2 schematically shows their cross-cutting nature. The subsequent chapters of this book describe the integrating mechanisms in detail.

"Guiding and tracking clients over time" refers to the fact that now, and even more so in the future, a person will select a single set of service providers (which may be linked through single ownership or merely

3

Figure 1-1.   Services of the Continuum of Care

Extended Care
Nursing facilities
Subacute
Nursing home follow-up
Swing beds
Hospice

Acute Care
Medical–surgical inpatient
Rehabilitation inpatient
Psychiatric inpatient
Consultation service
Interdisciplinary assessment unit

Ambulatory Care
Physicians' offices
Outpatient clinics
Community clinics
Assessment programs
Day hospitals
Adult day care centers
Sick-baby day care centers
Family counseling programs

Home Care
Medicare-certified home health agencies
Private home care agencies
Durable medical equipment
High technology home therapy
Hospice
Home visitors
Home delivered meals
Homemaker and personal care
Chore services
Caregivers
Respite
Money management

Outreach
Screenings and immunizations
Information and referral
Telephone contact
Emergency response systems
Transportation
Senior membership programs
Meals on wheels
Mobile vans
Health fairs
Ombudsman

Wellness
Patient and community education
Exercise classes
Recreation and social groups
Volunteers
Support groups
Congregate meals
Friendly visitors
Senior companions
Legal counseling

Housing
Independent senior housing
Continuing care retirement communities
Congregate care facilities
Assisted living facilities
Group homes

Note: Service is defined broadly. Each "service" may offer disease-specific or condition-specific care. For example, a home health agency may provide skilled nursing, social work services, or home health aide assistance; a nursing home may have an Alzheimer's unit, a rehabilitation unit, a ventilator unit; a medical–surgical service in an inpatient hospital may include a CCU or ICU.

Source: Evashwick, C. Definition of the continuum of care. In: C. Evashwick and L. Weiss, editors. *Managing the Continuum of Care*. Gaithersburg, MD: Aspen, 1987, p. 28. ©1987, Aspen Publishers, Inc. Reprinted with permission.

Figure 1-2.   Integrating Mechanisms

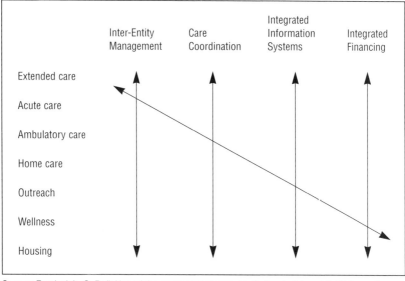

Source: Evashwick, C. Definition of the continuum of care. In: C. Evashwick and L. Weiss, editors. *Managing the Continuum of Care*. Gaithersburg, MD: Aspen, 1987, p. 25. ©1987, Aspen Publishers, Inc. Reprinted with permission.

formal affiliation) and probably a payer, and expect to stay with that system for an indefinite period of time for all of his or her health-related concerns. Wellness, as well as illness, will be the purview of health care providers, prompted by the financial incentives of managed care. Provider systems will want to attract clients, keep them healthy, and keep them in their system. This requires active and ongoing interaction and deliberate attempts to promote wellness rather than wait for illness.

A "comprehensive array of health, mental health, and social services" comprises the continuum. As the population ages, technology remedies or ameliorates acute problems, and chronic illness and disability dominate, increased attention must be paid to consumer demand for a holistic approach to care that includes mental well-being, social support, prevention, and wellness. In addition, families will want to belong to a system of care that meets the needs of all their members: children, parents, grandparents. The growth of managed care and the trend for employers to limit employee choices of insurance may further force families to select a single provider system with the expectation that it will meet the needs of all their members.

"All levels of intensity of care" reinforces the fact that the continuum recognizes that care for the chronically ill and health promotion for the healthy cannot succeed in isolation but, instead, require a spectrum of services, from the intensive medical care of the ICU to the nursing care of a skilled nursing facility (SNF) to the health promotion of a wellness program. The continuum of care concept is based on the premise that wellness/illness is multifaceted, and a piecemeal approach is inefficient and poor quality for the long term.

Underlying the concept of the continuum is the paradigm shift away from thinking of health care as "acute care" to recognizing that it should be ongoing, emphasizing wellness and accommodating chronic illness. The goal of health care is no longer only "cure" but is broadened to include prevention of illness, and for those who may already be ill, maintaining independence if cure is not possible. Measures of health status have expanded beyond clinical criteria to include functional status (that is, ability to perform the activities of daily living [ADL] and instrumental activities of daily living [IADL]) and prevention status (such as immunization status and lifestyle indicators). A comprehensive, integrated system of care encompasses the array of services a person needs over the course of a lifetime and coordinates those services to optimize use of individual, organizational, and societal resources. The ideal continuum will give its constituents access to the services they need whenever they need them, regardless of geographic location, financial status, or organizational auspices of the service.

Achieving "Seamlessness"

Achieving "seamlessness" is a difficult challenge that requires complex management. An organization need not own all the services of the continuum. Indeed, it is unlikely that any organization will be large enough to own all the services needed by all types of patients in all locations. Moreover, just because an organization has numerous services within its corporate umbrella or its affiliation network does not mean that those services are coordinated in a way that is either efficient for providers or easy for consumers. Thus, coordination and linkage among services becomes the challenge. No single model applies: Organizational forms from affiliations to ownership can work — or can be rampant with problems. Examples of multiple approaches exist, with successes and failures accompanying each. Each organization must create its own model based on its individual strengths and weaknesses, its community, its allies and competitors, and its target populations of potential users.

National statistics on the type and number of facilities and services reveal the way that availability limits creation of complete and discrete continuums of care blanketing the nation. Although not all statistics are precise, in round numbers, the U.S. has approximately 5,500 community hospitals,[2] 6,000 Medicare-certified home health agencies (about 1,200 of which are hospital based),[3] 6,000 private home care agencies,[4] 2,100 hospice programs,[5] 1,800 adult day care centers,[6] 15,000 nursing homes,[7] 650,000 physicians,[8] and 19,000 medical groups.[9] The uneven numbers of facilities, let alone their geographic locations, preclude a one-to-one match of services. In any given community, a service may be missing completely, be on the far side of town, have different operating auspices, or already be linked with a competitor.

From another perspective, except for very rural locations, most areas of the nation have a plethora of services. Indeed, many of today's health care systems, whether medical group based or hospital based, have an array of services within their corporation. However, linking the services in different combinations so that they meet the needs of individual patients is often problematic from the patient perspective. Managing the services so that they operate with a single purpose is equally challenging.

Manipulating the financing so that it enables comprehensive care rather than reinforcing fragmentation of care is yet another battle. Among the problems are historical fragmentation and individuality, much of which have grown out of separate financing streams and regulatory authorities. As the nation moves toward managed care with capitated financing and experiments with integrating the multiple financing streams of long-term care, the possibility exists that eventually the full continuum of acute and long-term care will be capitated, enabling providers to match services to need without external financial constraints. Funding for social support services could also be available and accessible through the health system. However, because the U.S. is not yet at the point of pooling financing streams, financing of the continuum must be creative, and financial barriers must be acknowledged and dealt with as effectively as possible.

Most of the services of the continuum of care have distinct characteristics. Each of the services on figure 1-1 can be characterized according to its target population, detailed types of services offered, staffing, governing and regulatory authorities, licensing and certification requirements, cost components, reimbursement methodologies, payer sources, geographic service area, capacity, availability, and measures of quality. The challenge of achieving uniform management can be envisioned by considering just one of these dimensions of the continuum.

The quality of care provided by a continuum should exceed that provided by a fragmented, uncoordinated set of services, and should be less costly due to being more efficient and less duplicative. In reality, there are little data on the effectiveness or efficiencies of the continuum, let alone its quality. Except for select demonstration projects, the continuum approach has not been widely tested or evaluated empirically. Measures of quality remain to be developed.

In brief, even getting all the service "pieces" of a continuum of care in place demands creativity. Managing those services as a single system, from the patient, provider, or payer perspective, is an achievement few have yet mastered!

Examples

Do seamless continuums of care exist? Two fictitious examples—Community Hospital and Comprehensive Cancer Center—illustrate the extremes of care within organizations that offer a wide range of services.

The Joneses' Experience with Community Hospital

Community Hospital's services include acute medical–surgical inpatient care, an emergency department (ED), a Medicare-certified home health agency affiliated through the hospital's parent corporation, a step-down unit, an adult day care center, an affiliated rehabilitation hospital also owned by the parent corporation, an ambulance company, a medical group of 200 physicians, and the usual complement of patient and family education.

When Mr. Jones suffers a stroke, his wife immediately calls the paramedics and their family physician. The ambulance takes him to Community Hospital because it is the closest ED. Because Mr. Jones's physician is out of town, the ED physician admits him to Community's medical unit. Mrs. Jones is not familiar with the hospital because she ordinarily uses another hospital in town. However, given that she cannot reach her husband's usual physician, and because of the distress caused by the immediate situation, she agrees to the admission. However, she has to search to find her husband's Medicare card. Because he has a permanent registration on file at the other hospital as well as at the physician's office, she has not used the card recently.

After four days of recuperation, the hospital suggests transferring Mr. Jones to its step-down unit. A different physician from the covering medical group has seen him each day, and because their regular physician is still out of town at a conference, Mrs. Jones complies. She has to go through the admitting process again because the step-down unit is technically a skilled nursing facility and requires its own admissions forms. Mr. Jones begins to receive physical therapy from the rehabilitation staff, but Mrs. Jones is advised to expect a separate bill for the rehabilitation services because they are technically contracted for from the medical group.

After 10 days, Mr. Jones is doing much better. He is medically stable, and the physician predicts near complete recovery assuming continued progress with rehabilitation. The physicians then recommend transferring Mr. Jones to the rehabilitation hospital affiliated with the hospital's parent corporation. Thus, he is transferred across town to a new hospital. Once again, Mrs. Jones must go through the admissions process, finding the Medicare card again and answering the same questions about address and next of kin. By now their regular physician has returned and comes to visit Mr. Jones. He tells Mrs. Jones that the care has been consistent with what he would have prescribed at their usual hospital. However, he tells her honestly that he will not be able to visit Mr. Jones daily in the rehabilitation hospital because it is so far across town; instead, he promises to monitor her husband's care weekly.

After three weeks at the rehabilitation hospital, Mr. Jones is declared well enough to go home and return for outpatient rehabilitation therapy. Because Mr. Jones may still be considered technically housebound, the discharge planner recommends at least one home visit by the home health agency. The physician and Mrs. Jones agree. Once again, Mrs. Jones must go through the admissions process with the home health agency. The nurse checks to ensure that Mr. Jones is maintaining his physical stability now that he is home, and helps arrange the house for the convenience of both Mr. and Mrs. Jones. However, she says that she will not be able to return because Mr. Jones appears to be on his way to recovery and does not have any problems legitimizing nursing attention. Mrs. Jones works part-time and cannot afford to quit her job. When she expresses concern about how her husband will manage when she is out of the house, the home care nurse suggests that he go to Community Hospital's day care center.

The following Monday, the Joneses go to the adult day care center where they once again must fill out admissions forms. They discover that, although the staff are very nice and Mr. Jones could be transported to the outpatient clinic for rehabilitation therapy, the majority of the people at the center suffer from Alzheimer's or some other form of dementia. Mr. Jones does not want to remain for the day, let alone return.

Mrs. Jones ends up taking a two-week leave of absence from work, hoping that her husband will be well enough to manage on his own after that. He decides to continue outpatient therapy at his original physician's hospital so that he can see his regular doctor more often and address the underlying medical conditions that caused the stroke. So, once more, the Joneses dig out their Medicare card and go through the admissions process. When they finally get to the clinic, they have to start from scratch to tell the therapist what happened, because no records have been transferred from the five other locations at which Mr. Jones has received care.

Meanwhile, at home, Mrs. Jones begins to receive bills from the hospital, the medical group, the ambulance company, the subacute nursing home, the home care agency, the rehabilitation therapists, their own physician, and the durable medical equipment company. She also receives five patient satisfaction questionnaires asking the Joneses to evaluate their experience.

Even though Community Hospital advertised that it offers a continuum of care, the experience of a single patient shows how disjointed care can be. Even if each individual provider offers the highest quality care, overall care is clearly inefficient and may even reduce quality due to the lack of communication among practitioners.

Mrs. Chen's Experience with Comprehensive Cancer Center

Comprehensive Cancer Center (CCC) does not advertise itself as offering a continuum of care. However, its motto is "to help our patients with whatever they need when they need it."

As part of a routine physical given by her internist, Mrs. Chen goes to CCC for an annual mammogram. The results indicate probable breast cancer, and the center sends them to Mrs. Chen's internist, asking whether he wants to contact his patient or whether he wants the CCC to contact her directly. Her internist opts to deliver the news to Mrs. Chen himself, but asks CCC to take over her care and to keep him informed.

The CCC assigns a nurse case manager to Mrs. Chen, who calls the patient later in the day after she has heard from her primary care doctor. The nurse asks Mrs. Chen to come in to meet with her and an oncologist and to arrange for a biopsy. When the nurse meets with Mrs. Chen, she advises her of support groups that she and her husband may wish to attend and also spends time with the patient telling her what to expect and helping her begin the treatment process, which she says may well last up to a year. When the biopsy confirms significant cancer, the oncologist calls Mrs. Chen with the news and asks her to come in to discuss treatment options.

After meeting with the oncologist, Mrs. Chen and her husband decide on radiation treatments, followed by surgery and then likely more radiation therapy. Throughout the entire process, the nurse case manager keeps in close touch with Mrs. Chen. She gives Mrs. Chen a beeper number that will enable her to reach the nurse at any time and arranges for Mrs. Chen to meet with a wig specialist at CCC one day each week to make a wig that will match Mrs. Chen's own hair. Mrs. Chen also meets with the CCC's nutritionist to make sure she follows the optimum diet.

Mrs. Chen knows that several physicians are involved with her treatment. There seem to be surgeons, and radiologists, and internists, and some others in white coats who manipulate the fancy equipment. They are all very nice. However, Mrs. Chen is also confident that a single oncologist is coordinating all this care at the physician level. In addition, she knows that he is keeping her own physician involved because she periodically receives a call from either her internist or his nurse to see if she has any problems she wants to discuss with them.

Immediately after surgery, Mrs. Chen is visited at home by a home care nurse whom she had met briefly at CCC prior to surgery. As promised, the nurse stopped in to see how Mrs. Chen was doing the day after she came home. The nurse seemed to know a lot about her condition, having spoken with the oncologist and the surgeon prior to the home visit.

For the most part, Mrs. Chen's care is covered by her HMO. However, she does have some copays to make and a few direct expenses. CCC has integrated all aspects of her care into a single bill, including the cost of the wig and support group contributions. The staff in CCC's resource office invite Mrs. Chen to sit down with them to go over her bill. They calculate for her exactly what she owes and explain each expense. Also, they enable her to make one check to CCC, and CCC assumes responsibility for paying each of the components. CCC also maintains a single record for Mrs. Chen. Regardless of which department/physician/provider was taking care of Mrs. Chen on a given day, the same purpose record kept showing up, and Mrs. Chen felt confident that the team was keeping track of what the others were doing on her behalf.

After a six-month process of active treatment, Mrs. Chen is declared on her way to recovery, with a good potential of no further medical problems due to the cancer. However, she is asked to return once a month for three months and then every three months for another year. She continues to meet with the support group, now sharing her experience with other newly diagnosed patients. The nurse calls her each month in between visits to see how she is doing. On her birthday, she receives a card from CCC celebrating another year of life. Mrs. Chen feels as though she has made close friends who care about her as well as for her. She feels that, no matter what she needed related to her cancer condition, the CCC staff could and would help her.

CCC functions as an exemplary continuum of care, addressing all aspects of a patient's physical and mental health condition, arranging access to a wide spectrum of services, and coordinating the care so that the patient does not have the sense of starting over again each time with a new set of providers and payers.

References

1. Evashwick, C. Definition of the continuum of care. In: C. Evashwick and L. Weiss, editors. *Managing the Continuum of Care.* Gaithersburg, MD: Aspen, 1987, p. 23.

2. American Hospital Association. *Annual Guide to Hospital Statistics.* Chicago, IL: AHA, 1995.

3. National Association of Home Care. *Basic Statistics About Home Care Facts, 1995.* Washington, DC: NAHC, 1996.

4. NAHC.

5. National Hospice Organization. *1994–95 Hospice Statistics*. Arlington, VA: NHO, 1995.

6. National Council on Aging. Direct communication with National Association of Adult Day Care Programs, Aug. 1996.

7. Cowles, C. M. *Nursing Home Statistical Yearbook*. Tacoma, WA: Cowles Research Group, Inc., 1995.

8. American Medical Association, Chicago, IL. Direct communication, Aug. 1996.

9. American Medical Association. *Medical Groups in the U.S., 1996*. Chicago: AMA, 1996.

Part Two

Operational Issues

Chapter 2

Consensus and Commitment

The first step in creating a continuum of care is an agreement among participating entities on an overarching vision of what they want to accomplish with a continuum. The goals for a continuum reflect, but differ from, the goals and objectives of individual participating entities.

Different entities may have different reasons for wanting to offer a seamless continuum of care: A managed care company may want to advertise a continuum in order to attract more members; a health care system may want to offer as many services as possible to maximize revenue streams; a physician organization may want to emphasize seamlessness in order to increase efficiencies and minimize expenses; or, a religious-based social service agency may want to offer a continuum for mission and quality imperatives. These differing goals may be compatible with the continuum's goals, but each of the participating entities should understand and accept the goals of the other individual entities. To implement the seamless continuum successfully, the participating entities must reach consensus upon the vision and goals for the continuum. Analyzing collective and individual goals at the outset of continuum formation and resolving inconsistencies early on will help to avoid operational conflicts that may occur later.

Organizational and individual priorities should also be recognized. Staff within each organization and colleagues of other collaborating organizations must also feel confident that the resources required for the continuum will be forthcoming based on the level of the board's and administration's commitment. An organization may believe in the continuum approach and may have goals that are consistent with it, but creating a continuum may not be a priority. For example, one hospital made a commitment to a continuum of care and hired a vice president to guide it, but the hospital was also engaged in a major renovation of the physical plant. The time and energy of staff throughout the hospital, as well as extra dollars, were devoted to the physical expansion. Although it was never formally stated, the reality was that any changes in service delivery processes or management structures and operations were deferred. The long-term commitment to creating a continuum was sincere, but the vice president was unable to get enough attention and resources to effect change because the continuum was simply not a priority.

Leadership is also essential in creating a continuum. Creating a continuum requires changing the way many providers and payers operate and think about health care. A seamless continuum of care depends on having leaders who understand the concept and are willing to support its implementation. The chief executive officer (CEO) and the board of each organization involved must be committed to the changes required to implement comprehensive, seamless care. Each organization also must have a top-level champion who can articulate the vision that will guide the organization's participation in creating the continuum and a senior administrator who has the authority to implement the needed changes (or who has the access to bring action issues to the attention of the CEO).

Following are the organizational tasks discussed in this chapter:

- Create a shared vision.
- Set goals and objectives.
- Identify committed leaders.
- Educate the board(s).
- Deal with organizations without boards similarly.
- Communicate with staff.

Create a Shared Vision

The service entities participating in the continuum should share a common vision of the desired patient, provider, and perhaps even payer, experience. A shared vision is particularly important when the continuum is a consortium or network model, or has many different component organizations, each with different goals and ways of measuring them. A shared vision will provide common ground for planning, implementing, and resolving differences. Without a common vision, it will be difficult to build compatible operations. The vision statement's ultimate focus should be on the patient rather than on the provider or payer. The process of creating a shared vision should include physicians and other clinicians as well as administrators. Figure 2-1 gives examples of vision statements of organizations that espouse a continuum of care approach.

Recommended Actions

- Create a continuum of care board or leadership advisory committee, including physicians and representatives of each of the major services involved.

Figure 2-1.   Example Mission and Vision Statements

Crozer-Keystone Health System

Created in 1989, Crozer-Keystone of Media, Pennsylvania, now encompasses three
acute care hospitals, five long-term care facilities, a managed care organization, a
primary care physician network, freestanding substance abuse centers, home health
agencies, and a multisite occupational health center.

> Crozer-Keystone Health System is committed to the improved health status of
> those persons we serve. Through a seamless, user-friendly continuum of quality
> health services including primary and health promotion, acute and long term
> care, through rehabilitative and restorative care, Crozer-Keystone will deploy its
> resources in a cost-effective and community-responsive manner. Working in
> partnership with our physicians and other health professionals, we will seek to
> forge new alliances with other community health and social service
> organizations. Working with our community, our goal is to build a healthy place
> to live and work and a sound environment in which to build and maintain our
> families.

Source: Crozer-Keystone Health System, Media, PA. Reprinted with permission.

Atlanta Senior Care

The Atlanta Senior Care, formed in late 1995, is a network of 14 care and service
organizations serving a senior adult population in Atlanta, with leadership provided by
Wesley Woods Geriatric Center at Emory University. Programs include: health
promotion and education; preventive health activities; congregate living centers;
primary medical care; acute care inpatient hospitals, including tertiary inpatient care;
outpatient and inpatient rehabilitation; inpatient and outpatient psychiatry; outpatient
geriatric specialty services; residential Alzheimer's program; intermediate care nursing
home; residential skilled nursing; home health, including skilled nursing, personal care,
and rehabilitation; residential hospice care; adult day care; senior centers; home meal
service; care management; and information and referral.

> The mission of Atlanta Senior Care is to "help senior adults maximize health and
> independence." The stated goal is "to integrate care and services across place,
> time and provider for senior adults and those who support them." The objective
> of Atlanta Senior Care is to develop an interdisciplinary network of care and
> service organizations to plan, provide and manage an array of health and
> support services to improve the quality of life of the senior population and their
> caregivers.

Source: Wesley Woods, Inc., Atlanta, GA. Reprinted with permission.

(Continued on next page)

Figure 2-1.   (Continued)

Loretto

Loretto, based primarily in Onondaga County, Central New York State, is in the process of transitioning from a loosely connected fee-for-service system into an integrated system of managed care. It includes a comprehensive array of housing options and community and residential-based health care services. Specifics include: four independent living facilities, seven supportive living facilities, assisted living, enriched housing, adult care programs, PACE (Program of All Inclusive Care for the Elderly), community residences for the developmentally disabled/mentally ill; three residential health care facilities; a health care diagnostic and treatment center; home care programs; adult medical day care programs, care planning, information and referral, home repair, transportation, respite care, emergency response systems, caregiving seminars.

> The mission of Loretto is to assist older adults and those with chronic health conditions to maintain their independence while offering opportunities to enrich their lives and maintain wellness.

Source: Loretto, Onondaga County, NY. Reprinted with permission.

The Bon Secours Health System—Richmond

Created in 1996, the Bon Secours Health System—Richmond comprises four acute care hospitals, geriatric assessment, retirement housing, a complete spectrum of home health services, a senior membership program, a skilled nursing transitional care unit, case management, 21 physician practices, comprehensive rehabilitation services, and a newly formed physician–hospital organization of 250 physicians.

> By the Year 2000, we will be the premier integrated health care delivery system in Central Virginia. Guided by our shared values and the needs of those we serve, each of us will act to set the quality standard for service to our community. As a leading integrated health system we will:
>
> • Establish partnerships with others to improve health
> • Develop service and programs in response to unmet needs
> • Develop systems for the coordination of patient services across a continuum of care
> • Create an environment that supports the development of people

Source: Bon Secours Health System, Richmond, VA. Reprinted with permission.

- Conduct a day-long retreat with the leaders of the participating entities to develop a common vision and to agree on goals and objectives, with written minutes of the retreat subsequently circulated to reinforce consensus.
- Publish a shared vision statement, listing all the participating entities to underscore their commitment to the continuum and their willingness to collaborate with each other.
- Field-test the vision with focus groups of consumers to obtain feedback, reinforcement, and direction for the participating entities.

Set Goals and Objectives

Each entity involved in creating a seamless continuum of care should articulate what it wishes to accomplish. General goals should be accompanied by specific, measurable objectives. Although there may be agreement on general goals, true congruence or real differences are likely to emerge when the evaluation criteria are explicit.

Figure 2-2 shows four main goals and companion objectives that have been found to be held by proponents of a seamless continuum of care. Most are compatible; however, in certain circumstances, goals may be contradictory. For example, an area lacking an adult day care center may advocate that such a service is important in offering clients access to a full range of services. The adult day care center would be consistent with goals of improving quality of care and meeting consumer demand. However, adult day care programs typically struggle to cover their costs. Unless external funding is readily available to support start-up and ongoing operations, opening an adult day care center is an expense incompatible with the goals of ensuring financial viability.

Recommended Actions

- Convene a senior management team representing the major participants of the continuum to develop a common set of goals and objectives. This may be a follow-up to an initial meeting devoted to articulating and gaining consensus on the vision.
- Have the partners in the continuum share the goals and objectives of their respective organizations, note their differences, and agree on a common set of goals and objectives.
- Alternatively, ask the management of each participating entity to prepare a separate statement of the goals and measurable objectives supporting its rationale for wanting to create a continuum of care. Goals should be shared and reviewed for compatibility.

Figure 2-2. Goals and Objectives of the Continuum of Care

1. To meet consumer demand
   a. To increase capacity to care for the growing population of chronically ill
   b. To reorient care to focus on chronic illness and functional ability
   c. To increase sensitivity to multidimensional—dimensional client needs
   d. To appeal to changing consumer preferences

2. To improve quality of care
   a. To provide comprehensive care, including wellness and prevention
   b. To provide continuity of care across sites and providers
   c. To develop collaborative relationships with community agencies
   d. To optimize use of advanced technologies
   e. To deal with patient rights and ethical issues

3. To ensure financial viability
   a. To prepare for managed care financing, including capitation
   b. To maximize payment for care
   c. To generate new revenue streams
   d. To offset fixed overhead
   e. To spread or minimize risk
   f. To gain economies of scale
   g. To gain greater access to capital
   h. To improve efficiency of operations

4. To enhance market position
   a. To compete for managed care contracts
   b. To compete for managed care enrollees
   c. To capture new clients
   d. To enter new markets
   e. To enhance financial competitiveness
   f. To attract physicians, payers, and other strategic partners
   g. To outpace competing organizations

Source: Updated from C. Evashwick and L. Weiss, editors. *Managing the Continuum of Care.*
Gaithersburg, MD: Aspen, 1987, p. 86. ©1987, Aspen Publishers, Inc. Reprinted with permission.

Identify Committed Leaders

A continuum of care needs both administrative and clinical leaders, including physicians, who understand and espouse the continuum's vision. This is imperative to gaining board and physician support for and staff loyalty to the concept. Leaders also must have the necessary authority, or access to those with authority, to implement the continuum's concepts. Having the availability of leadership may mean establishing formal positions and paying clinicians and/or administrators to devote the time to the continuum that it requires. To plan the continuum of care for the Chicago area, for example, Lutheran General HealthSystem (now Advocate Health Care) organized a team of senior administrators who agreed to devote their energies full-time to the project for an entire year, relinquishing their regular jobs to others. The fact that senior staff would take on the job, and that the system would establish special positions for a year for them to do so, indicated the system's level of commitment to the continuum.

Recommended Actions

- Establish the position of director of the continuum of care with a title and locus within the organization that signifies the continuum's importance. If multiple entities are involved and each designates a continuum representative, stature and authority within each entity should be comparable (if not identical in title).
- Create a senior management committee of directors (of the participating entities) whose function it is to handle the political aspects of the continuum and to provide executive direction and decision making within their own organization.
- Establish an advisory committee of representatives of departments, community agencies, and consumers who may not have formal roles in the continuum as service providers, but who are stakeholders in the continuum.
- Appoint a physician director of the continuum of care. Ideally, he or she would be the medical director of a nursing home or home health agency, as well as a prominent and respected member of the hospital's medical staff and the medical group or greater physician community.
- Create a task force of staff to address clinical delivery and support operations and work with the continuum director to plan and implement the continuum. Representatives should have authority within the unit they represent.
- Include physicians on the continuum of care task force charged with planning and developing the continuum.
- Give visibility to continuum leaders in internal and community-oriented publications.

Educate the Board(s)

Typically, boards have responsibility for the governance of one or more of the specific services comprising the continuum of care. Except for a few innovative organizations that have created continuum boards, most boards have been convened and run to serve a more limited entity. Because some boards may be uncomfortable with their organization embarking on new dimensions of care, they need to be educated about what a continuum of care is, why it is important, and what the implications are for operations, quality of care, financial status, and market position. Each of the organizations involved in the continuum will need to bring its board along.

Recommended Actions

- Include members of the board on the continuum of care management or advisory committees.
- Develop and conduct educational programs to be presented to the board of each of the participating entities.
- Convene joint meetings of the boards of the participating entities so that they can share common education/information and get to know one another.
- Educate foundation boards as well as governing boards.
- Ask what types and frequency of reports the boards want to receive and report regularly so that board involvement and education are ongoing.

Deal with Organizations without Boards Similarly

Many health care organizations do not have traditional boards. For example, for-profit entities may be dealing with shareholders and a board whose members have individual financial ties with the company. Many individual and family-owned businesses are found in the home health and nursing home arenas. Government entities, such as public health departments and the local Area Agency on Aging, may have informal advisory committees but no official board. A huge bureaucracy can make identifying decision makers quite challenging. Alternatively, persuading family members to be of a common mind can be equally challenging. For-profit companies may face difficulties in having one member committed to the vision of a continuum and yet be outvoted by others. Whatever the legal structure, it is imperative to identify those individuals having authority to make decisions and to commit the organization to collaborative arrangements. Deal with them in the same way as boards—involve, educate, and communicate.

Recommended Actions

- Identify leaders and visionaries for each participating entity.
- Identify those in each participating entity who have authority to commit the organization.

- Meet with each person of vision and authority for each participating entity, and find out what his or her personal vision and goals are for the organization and how the continuum helps accomplish them.
- Develop informational/educational materials, marketing materials, and persuasion statements appropriate for the particular governance structures of each of the entities participating in the continuum.

Communicate with Staff

The vision and its accompanying mission statement must be verbalized and communicated so that everyone who is part of the continuum and its affiliated components understands what the continuum is about and why it is important. Staff at all levels of all the participating entities should know about the continuum of care, including the vision, the goals and objectives, and the evaluation criteria. They should understand the day-to-day implications for both them and the patients/clients with whom they interact. As many communication vehicles as possible should be used, and communication about the continuum should be ongoing.

Recommended Actions

- Conduct an all-staff orientation meeting on the continuum for each participating entity.
- Incorporate information about the continuum as part of regular staff meetings.
- Clearly articulate goals and objectives in writing to all staff. This may be in the form of a one-page vision statement, an article in the organization's newsletter, a flyer enclosed in pay vouchers, and any other written communication vehicle used by the organizations.
- Have each department or subunit involved with the continuum devote a staff meeting or special time to understanding what its purpose is, what different actions it might require on their part, and how to explain it to patients.
- Develop a way to exchange information with service partners on a regular basis aimed at reinforcing the continuum concept to the staff of all participating entities. For example, include a monthly "continuum of care" column in your own newsletter and invite key members of affiliated services to guest-write it.

Chapter 3

Patient/Client Focus

A seamless continuum of care that integrates all services and guides and tracks clients over time through periods of both illness and wellness is the ideal for all people. However, patients differ in service use patterns, and organized continuums are *most* cost-effective for those needing complex services over an extended period of time. Once an organization has established a continuum for one population, the lessons and the operating systems are more readily transferable to another population.

Although not every patient will use every service, common patterns are likely among patients with similar conditions. Table 3-1 shows examples of continuum services likely to be used by patients with two different conditions. Especially when first striving for a seamless continuum of care, it is more effective to identify a select target audience and organize around the needs of a particular type of patient rather than all patients. Examples of patients who would benefit most from a seamless continuum of care include: people suffering from cancer; recent stroke victims; people needing rehabilitation after acute trauma, stroke, fracture, or other conditions; people with prolonged mental health needs; pregnant women; older people with complex mental and/or physical conditions; children with congenital abnormalities and their families; anyone with multiple chronic conditions and/or functional disabilities. The systems and procedures established in creating one continuum can later be expanded to apply to other populations.

Organizations offering many services under the corporate umbrella may tout their "continuum of care," when, in reality, their services are coordinated at neither the individual patient nor the administrative level and, despite appearances, are insufficient to meet the needs of any particular type of patient. Focusing on a specific target population enables the organization to develop a patient-oriented system of care. Rather than building a system based on administrative expedience, the continuum is built around the needs of patients. Thus, in the long run, it is likely to be a more effective and more efficient system of care.

Table 3-1.   Example Continuums of Care for Select Target Populations: Contrast in Service Components

Services	Target Populations	
	Cancer Patients	**Alzheimer's**
Inpatient hospital	Surgery	Not necessary
Outpatient	Radiation therapy Chemotherapy Rehabilitation	Specialty assessment clinic Adult day care Monitor medical conditions
Patient education	Cancer-specific	Oriented toward families and care-givers
	Special adaptations (e.g., wigs, prostheses) Cancer-specific support	Caregiver support group
Home health	Nursing visits Home infusion therapy for chemotherapy Hospice	Friendly companion Respite relief Homemaker
Patient care team	Medical oncologists Surgical oncologists Radiation oncology team	Geriatrician Geriatric social worker Nurse practitioner Case manager
Counseling	(Potential) bereavement counseling Estate Planning Funeral planning Nutrition counseling	Caregiver counseling Home modification Consultation
Follow-up and wellness	Periodic call to patient and family to check status at 3, 6, 9, 12 months	Immunization check Physical activity

Note: The services cited above may be provided by separate and/or numerous entities.

A guiding principle of the continuum of care is that it is client oriented, meaning that it is designed to meet the patient's needs rather than those of the payer or provider. Furthermore, the continuum definition assumes that the patient will be with the system for an indefinite period of time. This warrants a holistic approach to the patient as a person, including consideration of family, support system, living arrangements, housing conditions, economic status, ethnic background, religious preferences. All of these spheres affect a person's health over the long term. Thus, these multiple facets should be considered in providing each specific service. In addition, they may offer insights about additional services that should be coordinated for a given individual.

For example, an appropriate support system may be the single greatest factor determining whether a patient can remain at home after a debilitating stroke. Here is an example of how this can work. Mr. Lee and Mrs. Fernandez both had strokes on the same day. Mr. Lee had a devoted and able spouse who could help with his daily rehabilitation exercises and otherwise manage home and financial affairs. Conversely, Mrs. Fernandez was a widow who lived alone and had no children. When the hospital social worker learned that Mrs. Fernandez was an active member of a local church, she talked to the minister, who was able to mobilize a group of women to help with Mrs. Fernandez's care at home by providing visitation, meals, transportation, and assistance with activities of daily living. The physician was then able to order home health care with the confidence that his patient was not in jeopardy by returning home. In this instance, the church was a key participant in the patient's continuum of care. Rather than just considering the services that were formal members of the organization's network of affiliates, the physician and the social worker took a holistic approach to determining what the patient's needs and resources were.

Following are the patient/client focus tasks discussed in this chapter:

- Select a target population.
- Create a patient care task force.
- Characterize the patient population's special needs.
- Delineate patient flow, current and ideal.
- Educate staff and providers about target populations served.
- Educate patients and families.
- Deal with dual diagnoses.

Select a Target Population

As noted above, continuums are most effectively initiated by organizing around the needs of a specific target population, particularly one including patients with multifaceted conditions (and hence users of multiple services) and conditions likely to last over time. The criteria may be a particular diagnosis (for example, congestive obstructive pulmonary disease [COPD], AIDS) or several diagnoses using the same services (for example, rehabilitation patients). High-risk groups most likely to benefit from a continuum of care include people with congestive heart failure, COPD, diabetes, cancer, stroke, or Alzheimer's. However, there are a number of other factors that may be involved in the selection of a target population. For example, the organization just beginning to move toward a seamless system of care may choose to start with a relatively small population with discrete needs and thus limit the number of staff and services involved in implementing its pilot continuum. Alternatively, the organization intending to make creation of the continuum a top priority and to devote a wealth of resources to the necessary changes may choose to start with its highest-volume patient group. The organization's particular goals in creating a continuum also may affect its selection of a target population, as may the organization's size. Small organizations may choose a broader target population than large organizations with high volumes of many types of patients.

Recommended Actions

- Articulate criteria for selecting a patient population consistent with the organization's goals for creating a continuum.
- Identify potential target populations.
- Characterize each target population according to volume, payment, geographic location, and other factors.
- Examine competition to determine who else serves this target population; verify that a viable market exists.
- Examine community agencies that provide complementary services to the target population and that may be potential collaborators or referral sources.
- Conduct focus groups of potential patients and families to get input on service needs, care dilemmas, and preferences for care delivery.
- Select the target population to be the focus of the continuum, delineating eligibility criteria acceptable and understandable to participating entities.

Create a Patient Care Task Force

The task force convened to plan the care continuum, and the ongoing management team should include physicians and other clinicians (see chapter 5). In addition, a subgroup or additional task force may be warranted during initial planning or periods of major expansion to focus on clinical issues. Inclusion of physicians, nurses, social workers, and therapists will ensure that a continuum is designed that provides high-quality care (rather than one that meets administrative criteria but falls short of optimal care from the clinical or patient perspective). Clinical team composition will vary depending upon the patient population. For example, an interdisciplinary team focused on people with mental illness may emphasize the need to include the nurse at the employer's health clinic, whereas a team focused on people with Alzheimer's disease may include a social worker who leads a support group offered by the Alzheimer's Association. The clinical task force can be given responsibility for accomplishing tasks delineated below.

Recommended Actions

- Convene a patient-oriented continuum of care planning team that includes clinicians representing each participating entity, physicians, and an array of other disciplines.
- Identify individuals in the community who might be part of the team (clinicians from community agencies or savvy consumers).
- Select a physician and a clinician to champion the cause and gain widespread clinical support for the continuum for the particular target population.
- Identify existing clinical guidelines or protocols and measures of quality that apply to the target population.

Characterize the Patient Population's Special Needs

Once a target population is identified, its service needs must be cataloged and the source of those services delineated. Many services will exist within the organization participating in the continuum of care; others may be in the community. Either way, issues in coordination cannot be identified until a comprehensive list of services has been compiled. Services should be characterized according to availability and accessibility (including sources of reimbursement and eligibility requirements), and also for quality. This detailed analysis will reveal that some services that indeed exist in the organization (or in the community) are not applicable to the target population. For example, an organization may have its own home health agency, but in designing a continuum for high-risk pregnancy and newborns, the home health agency that specializes in home apnea monitoring and neonatal home care may be the competitor's. Or a social worker in the community with an excellent reputation for guiding Alzheimer's support groups may welcome a few patients/families from the continuum but not be willing to work for the continuum exclusively. One community hospital decided to develop a continuum of care for older patients that included a rehabilitation program but found that, despite the fact that it had a 25-person staff, the center staff specialized in sports medicine. No one in the rehab department had either the time or inclination to care for geriatric stroke victims.

In an era of increasing cultural diversity, sensitivity to ethnic and cultural preferences, as well as awareness of the concomitant resources available throughout the community, is yet another aspect of assessing patient need. Those from different ethnic groups may have service preferences unique to their culture.

Recommended Actions

- Delineate the services needed by the typical target population of patients and families from the clinicians' perspective.
- Convene a focus group of target population patients and families to find out what services they have used; what services they like; and what problems they have experienced in access, cultural sensitivity, availability, and coordination.
- Identify the services available to the target population within both the continuum entities and the community.
- Compare needed services with availability, identify gaps and opportunities, and plug this information into the service planning tasks described in chapter 4.

Delineate Patient Flow, Current and Ideal

Once services have been identified and their sources delineated, actual patient flow should be mapped. This will provide a revelation regarding the extent of seamlessness from the patient's perspective. Mapping lays the groundwork for setting up the integrating mechanisms that are the essence of having a seamless system of care rather than a set of fragmented services advertised as a continuum. It also will show the relationships between services available within the continuum and those available externally.

Recommended Actions

- Map typical patient flow, including dimensions such as location, authorizations, record focus and format, and key staff responsible.
- Map ideal patient flow, including the same dimensions mentioned above.
- Save these maps because they can be used for other tasks of the continuum, such as formulating the management structure for the continuum, setting up the case management system, and evaluating progress.

Educate Staff and Providers about Target Populations Served

Some continuums of care receive wide attention; others are basically ignored. Physicians, other providers, and staff need to know what target populations an organization serves with its continuum. For example, a community hospital recently spent two months and many dollars publicizing its new cancer center, culminating in a week of grand openings for various audiences. In contrast, its existing continuum of care for geriatric patients was given no visibility. The geriatrics program offices were off-site, and many of the program's services were either community or outpatient based, rather than inpatient based. As a result, the cancer center received referrals from all of the hospital's physicians whereas referrals to the geriatrics program came mostly from community agencies and patient word of mouth. Although the health care system was located in an area heavily populated by older people, it lost many potential clients looking for a seamless continuum of care because it failed to educate its own referral network about its service continuum.

Recommended Actions

- Incorporate a presentation about the continuum and its target market into regularly scheduled staff meetings of participating entities.
- Hold special staff education sessions to describe the continuum, the target market, and how staff and patients access the continuum.
- Feature the continuum and a patient/family served by it in in-house news bulletins and publications.
- Create a regular "continuum patient of the month" feature for newsletters and establish a photo site to display the patient's/family's picture.
- Inform physicians about the continuum and explain how to identify and refer patients from the target population. Present at regular medical staff meetings or conduct a special grand rounds as a way of demonstrating how the continuum works and how it helps a typical patient from the target group.

Educate Patients and Families

Continuum of care is a term that is unlikely to mean much to most patients and families. Yet it is important that the people for whom the continuum is being created understand how to access it, how it works, and what advantages it offers them. In particular, they need to know that the continuum is designed specifically for people with their special needs. Creating awareness among and demand by consumers will help increase use and thus reinforce the continuum's value to its participating entities.

Recommended Actions

- Develop a brochure aimed at the specific target audience and make it available through each of the participating entities.
- Conduct invitational programs to inform potential users about the continuum.
- Conduct a well-publicized opening, with press, pictures, and refreshments.
- Develop a volunteer program specifically for the continuum and engage the volunteers in publicizing the program to their friends, family, and community.
- Reach out to potential users at sites where they are likely to be found (for example, sponsor a luncheon about the geriatrics continuum at the local senior center).
- Incorporate patient/family evaluation criteria that focus on the continuum into routine patient evaluation questionnaires—that is, ask consumers if the continuum works for them and how it differs from less organized care.

Deal with Dual Diagnoses

Organizations that create or participate in several continuums eventually will face the dilemma of a patient who qualifies for more than one—for example, a stroke victim with Alzheimer's who might be appropriate for either a rehabilitation continuum or an Alzheimer's continuum, or a patient with COPD who also is diagnosed with cancer. Which continuum is appropriate? Ultimately, a health care organization should be set up to manage all of its patients with a continuum of care approach. A case manager or a triage intake coordinator from one continuum should be able to use the integrated information system to link the patient with services accessed through any continuum. However, in the developmental stages, this is not done easily, and even once established, continuity of care will be maximized only if the patient and family are linked with one interdisciplinary team and/or one case manager. In the first example above, the patient may be set up with the continuum most appropriate for an immediate need, such as stroke rehabilitation for three months, then switched over to the Alzheimer's continuum for long-term management. The continuums may be operated by the same organization or network of organizations, or may be operated by entirely distinct organizations, in which case turf and payment issues may arise. Situations also may arise in which two members of a family are involved in different continuums—for example, a wife with cancer and a husband with Alzheimer's. This is not necessarily a problem, but coordination among the case managers or other clinicians arranging care for each patient is needed to ensure that each patient is being dealt with within the complete context of the home and social support situation.

Recommended Actions

- Identify patients that frequently overlap or are appropriate for more than one continuum and look for patterns in use and problems in the existing process.
- Bring staff of different continuums together periodically to discuss issues in common, how the continuums are different, and how care can be coordinated.
- Develop policies and procedures for transferring patients from one continuum to another.
- Incorporate questions into the patient evaluation form that will identify confusion, duplication of effort, and smooth transitions.

Chapter 4

Services of the Continuum

As mentioned in chapter 1, a comprehensive continuum of care that meets both the health and related social support needs of a particular individual may require as many as 50 different services to manage care over time. (See figure 1-1.) It is unlikely that any single organization will be able to own all these services (at least in the near future under the extant government and insurance systems). Moreover, even the services that an organization does own may not serve all the organization's patients due to any number of individual factors such as geography, specialty needs, patient preference, reimbursement, and so on. Thus, organizations constructing continuums should create systems that are flexible enough to meet the needs of individual patients and still meet the overall goal of creating a single, seamless system of care.

Although the services identified in chapter 1 are likely to be relevant to a large number of patients, different services will be used by different patient groups and used in different amounts. For example, an obstetrics continuum should include prenatal visits to physicians and nurse practitioners, labor and delivery at a hospital, home care, perhaps child care, family-oriented education, and access to counseling. For this continuum, buying a nursing home or setting up an adult day care center would be totally irrelevant. In contrast, however, the continuum for stroke patients might include the hospital, internist and neurologist offices, a rehabilitation unit, a skilled nursing facility (SNF), a step-down unit, home care, outpatient therapies (at a comprehensive outpatient rehabilitation facility [CORF], outpatient center, or physician's office), patient education, meals-on-wheels, adult day care, and aging network programs. Therefore, from the point of view of patients, it makes sense to develop a seamless system of care around their needs and not for administrative convenience.

Once the basic integrating mechanisms (shown in figure 1-2) are in place and precedent is set for structures and governance, expansion to other populations can occur. Similarly, once formal or informal relationships have been established with other providers in the community, those providers can be drawn on to serve the needs of additional populations.

Are Centers of Excellence continuums of care? Not necessarily. The Center of Excellence concept was popular among hospitals in the mid-1980s as a way of grouping services together to market to a designated audience, such as women, cancer patients, and sports medicine patients. Whatever it may be called in the 1990s, a Center of Excellence may indeed have an array of services that are all potentially appropriate for patients with a certain condition or other features in common. However, the ideal continuum deliberately links services; is likely to have a single individual responsible for shepherding the patient through the service options (for example, a case manager, the leader of an interdisciplinary team); assumes responsibility for wellness, prevention, and maintenance, as well as episodic care; has a comprehensive and integrated patient record; extends beyond the organization into the community when needed services are not available internally; and, ultimately, has control over payment. Thus, an existing Center of Excellence may provide a good base for a continuum but must be evaluated to determine what actions are needed for it to evolve it into a continuum. Similarly, product-line or service-line organizations provide a basis on which to develop a continuum but alone are not equivalent to a seamless continuum of care.

As noted in chapter 1, each service is likely to have its own operating characteristics. These must be thoroughly understood, and management and patient care organized to balance meeting patient need with accepting service constraints.

Following are the continuum services tasks discussed in this chapter:

- Determine which services to include.
- Assess existing services.
- Assess services for fit.
- Deal with split loyalties.
- Plan to fill service gaps.
- Handle service duplication.

Determine Which Services to Include

The services to be included in the continuum depend on the target population. (See chapter 2.) Service articulation requires a thorough understanding of the target population and thus follows the tasks outlined in chapter 2. Service availability, accessibility, and quality affect the management structure a continuum will use to develop its service package (for example, through affiliation, purchase, joint venture). The Sisters of

Providence in Alaska convened a task force comprising the CEOs of the hospital, nursing home, home health agency, outpatient rehabilitation center (CORF), and senior housing complex. Although all were affiliated in some way with the corporate office, each was an independent corporation. Collectively, they examined the continuum of care for those needing skilled nursing, intermediate care, subacute care, and assisted living. They determined service gaps and duplications and then formulated a plan to structure a collaborative continuum of care for those needing long-term care. Similarly, the former Sisters of Charity of Cincinnati developed Continuum of Care Task Forces at each of its major hospitals to look specifically at geriatric services.

Recommended Actions

- Convene a task force of clinicians and administrators to ascertain what services a typical patient of the target population needs over time. Depending on the size and scope of services of your own organization, the task force may include just representatives of internal services or both internal and other services in the community. Eventually, services external to the initiating organization are likely to be included.
- Survey former or potential patients to determine from their perspective what services they need or use. Seek out and review any recent market research done by any of the individual services, community agencies, or by commercial marketing firms.
- Select a sample of typical patients and have staff determine what services they used during an episode of illness, being sure to include services from within the organizations and outside. (This builds on the patient flow mapping mentioned in chapter 3.)
- Invite a group of community leaders and stakeholders to share their opinions about what services are needed for the continuum and how they see their organizations fitting in.
- In anticipation of managed care, evaluate services required of health plans for licensure.
- Review recent literature on outcomes research pertaining to each service.
- After a complete list of services is developed, prioritize them according to those that are essential and those that can be added in phases.
- Assess all services for reimbursement potential.

Assess Existing Services

Assuming that a list of the ideal services of the continuum has been developed, existing services must be evaluated for their fit into the desired continuum. All services should be available, accessible, and provide high-quality care.

Some services may not be available or accessible. For example, there are only about 1,800 formal adult day care centers and 2,100 formal hospices in the entire United States. The service may simply not be available in the continuum's geographic area. Even if services are available, they may not be accessible for a variety of reasons: they may be at capacity, may be affiliated with a competitor, may have religious affiliations that limit their applicability to all patients, may be difficult to access due to geographic location or the physical plant, or may have limited operating hours.

Quality is the third criterion on which services must be evaluated. Despite all the work that has been and is being done on quality and outcomes measures, the attention has been primarily on acute care. For some of the services of the continuum, standardized measures of quality outcomes have not yet been developed or uniformly adopted. Thus, the task force developing the continuum should specify criteria for quality for each service, then measure each of the existing services by those criteria to the extent that data can be obtained. Quality measures may be both objective and subjective, and they may be patient, provider, and payer perceptions.

Recommended Actions

- Identify and map existing services, including details about hours of operation, location(s), and financial and other criteria affecting patient acceptance. This may be done by the organization's planning department (if one exists), a consultant, or an intern or administrative staff member. The task force can help in the initial identification of services, but compiling complete and parallel information is more readily accomplished if assigned to one person.
- Develop criteria for accessibility and quality. These may be done by a task force or by administrators of various services who know the data and measures used in each field. Senior management of each service also may have input on criteria.
- Evaluate each service, both internal and external, using the criteria for availability, accessibility, and quality. The resulting product should produce decision-making information about service gaps and potential partners.

Assess Services for Fit

Whether services are within the same organization or are being added through affiliation, purchase, or other means, the continuum needs to determine whether indeed the service fits. Factors to be examined include characteristics of the populations served, geographic area served, culture, management capabilities, clinical capabilities, operating systems, and accreditation standards. Some of the characteristics may be revealed during the initial analysis; others will only become known through more in-depth exploration. One multi–health care system bought an SNF to take its Medicaid patients out of the hospital. However, the SNF had a patient population that was 90 percent private pay. Although the physical plant and license were a match, the facility had to completely change its marketing, staff orientation, and expectations about its bottom line. Incorporating the SNF into the hospital's continuum turned out to be much more problematic than anticipated. More careful up-front analysis would have helped both organizations to plan and implement the collaborative relationship more smoothly.

Recommended Actions

- Establish criteria for the entities that will participate in the continuum.
- Evaluate corporate culture, vision, and mission.
- Gather and compare significant operating policies and procedures, such as admission, discharge, and transfer policies.
- Conduct focus groups in the community and/or of potential users to learn their perceptions of the various entities potentially participating in the continuum.
- Acquire market research that may have been done for other reasons that reveals market share and consumer perceptions.

Deal with Split Loyalties

In trying to put the entire continuum together, an organization may identify a service in the community with which it would like to affiliate, but the service may be one component of a larger organization with which the first organization does not wish to affiliate. For example, a hospital may contract with a home health agency for its hospice program because it is the only one in town, but contract with a different home health agency for the majority of its business. Can this arrangement be negotiated and sustained over time? Will one or the other agency demand 100 percent of the hospital's business? Will staff know when to call which agency? What happens if a patient referred to the hospice home health agency changes his or her mind but still needs home health care? Does the patient stay with the agency from which he or she first received service or switch to the other agency?

Two large hospital systems in Southern California that owned hospitals serving adjacent areas merged to strengthen their position as providers. However, each owned a health maintenance organization (HMO), and the two HMOs served similar clients in overlapping areas. In putting together a geriatric continuum, one of the hospitals negotiated a superior senior product with one of the HMOs. This resulted in a change of enrollment for seniors from one HMO to the other and a subsequent shift in use from one hospital to the one with the geriatrics program. The hospital with the geriatric continuum succeeded in capturing market share and generating more revenue, but the harmony between hospital and health plan administrators within the new combined corporation suffered. Advance discussions and corporate policies may not have changed the contracts, but may have assuaged the negative interpersonal rivalry.

Recommended Actions

- Anticipate the issue of split loyalties (especially in affiliation agreements) and clearly articulate the conditions and directions of patient referral.
- Develop clear internal operating policies about patient referrals.
- Educate all staff about the possible problems in referrals, inform them of institutional policies, and let them know how to handle patients, families, and providers appropriately.
- Educate patients and families in advance about the directions and reasons for referrals.
- Through negotiations done at the corporate level, recognize the strengths and weaknesses of each service and project performance based on contribution to the continuum, even if that contribution is one of relinquishing business to a competing service.
- Through a case manager, primary care physician, information system, or other mechanism, stay in touch with a patient if he or she is indeed referred to services with which your organization does not have an exclusive referral agreement.
- Maintain communication with service competitors; affiliations and referral patterns may shift in the future.

Plan to Fill Service Gaps

Examining the services available for a target population may reveal that services designed to meet its specific needs are not available, even if a more generic service exists. For example, adult day care may be available in the community but may be a social model that does not offer health care, or alternatively, it may be a health-oriented day care program that limits the number of Alzheimer's patients it will accept. Only when services are examined specific to a target population can such gaps be identified. The organization must then decide how to fill the gaps. Options include purchasing, starting, affiliating, joint venturing, or (and this is often the most challenging) revamping an existing service to participate as part of the continuum. Structure is discussed in more detail in chapter 5.

Recommended Actions

- Assess the resources available from all the services potentially participating in the continuum to determine what personnel, space, capital, and so on can be contributed to develop the needed service. Look for excess capacity that could be put to good use, but do not force inappropriate relationships.
- Consult legal counsel for legal and regulatory factors that determine or limit options.
- Analyze managed care arrangements for their effect on service affiliations.
- Clearly state goals and objectives of the anticipated continuum in any deals that involve purchase, merger, joint venture, affiliation, or start-up done by contract. All added services must understand the goals of the continuum, and be willing and able to comply with the operational implementation of a continuum.
- Designate a single administrator or task force member responsible for delineating the administrative options for adding each service to the continuum. If too many administrators are making too many different deals, using different criteria, and conveying different goals, the continuum may end up with a potpourri of relationships and myriad expectations that confuse rather than streamline patient care.
- Develop a plan for adding the missing services that articulates capital requirements and phasing as necessary.

Handle Service Duplication

In assessing the services required for a continuum, an organization may discover that, rather than a gap, its continuum has several potential sites for certain types of care. In moving toward a comprehensive continuum approach, which service does it include? Does it deliberately exclude services, particularly if it owns them or has a close affiliation with them? If overall demand in the community is sufficient, each of the services may be operating at or near full capacity. However, the organized continuum of care approach may alter existing referral patterns and result in one service losing business to the point that it loses financial viability.

The Sisters of Providence Alaska Continuum of Care Task Force, mentioned above, found that all five organizations participating on the task force served adults with long-term functional disabilities. However, the total demand for such services was less than the total capacity of the combined organizations. The five participating entities agreed to certain criteria that would direct patients to one of the five specific providers *and* agreed that duplication would prevail: they would continue to compete for the more general long-term care patient.

Home health is a common example of when duplication is likely to occur. Approximately one-third of hospitals own or have in their corporation a home health agency. Many medical groups also have their own home care agencies. With the rash in recent years of hospital–hospital mergers and medical group–hospital mergers, duplication can be expected. Over time, two agencies may be combined, but in the short term, which one gets the referrals? These occurrences of duplication should be recognized by all entities potentially participating in the continuum and discussed frankly, and consensus should be reached as to how to handle them with fairness to all involved, including the patient and family.

Recommended Actions

- Clearly identify service duplication in terms of specific services provided and population served.
- Work with the duplicative services to gain agreement on the criteria for referral, distinguishing referrals if possible.
- Formulate explicit policies for referrals (for example, according to geography or specialty service; or simply alternate).
- Communicate referral policies and procedures to staff, particularly the staff doing triage and referral.
- Monitor the performance of both services to ensure equal quality and compliance with the agreed-upon referral process.
- Incorporate patient choice and continuity of patient care into referral criteria.

Chapter 5

Structure and Management

Once the services of a continuum have been identified and the participating entities have agreed in principle to work together to provide a seamless continuum of care, the organizations involved must determine how they are going to structure their relationship. Two elements are important: how the services are formally structured for legal and reimbursement purposes, and how they work on a day-to-day basis. A seamless continuum of care is more than just a collection of services in that services are actively coordinated, not just available. Patients are followed over time, with the service configuration changed as their needs change; and services throughout the community are incorporated through integrating mechanisms (for example, the case management for the continuum arranges for meals-on-wheels from the Area Agency on Aging and includes this in the patient's record).

How services are structured depends at least in part on ownership: Are all services part of the same parent corporation? (Just because they are does not mean that they will automatically be seamless.) Is each service independent? Are the services component parts of different parent corporations? The variations are endless—and thus, so are the organizational configurations. History and culture affect how an organization is structured, as do legal, tax, and financial considerations. In addition, similar organizations based in different states may have different structures due to the constraint of state laws. One state allows physicians to be corporate employees; but another requires a physician–hospital organization (PHO) structure within which to transact hospital–physician joint enterprise business as "arm's-length transactions" to comply with Medicare fraud and abuse and corporate practice of medicine statutes. The technical legal and financial considerations are beyond the scope of this book, and it is strongly recommended that organizations seek expert advice from lawyers, accountants, and other appropriate professionals. However, a number of operational issues apply regardless of the legal and financial issues that guide structure.

At least three levels of structure are relevant to managing a continuum. First, each individual service that is part of the continuum must be structured internally to participate as part of an overall system rather than as a discrete service. Throughout this book these services are referred to as "participating entities" because their organizational status may range from being a discrete organization to being a department within an organization that is in turn part of a larger corporation. Within a single service, clinicians' and administrators' tasks will change from being insular to externally focused, and job descriptions, performance expectations, and operating procedures will be changed to reflect the differences. For example, a social work department that formerly kept records of discharges according to generic categories, such as nursing homes and home health agencies, revised its referral procedures and record keeping to emphasize discharges to the nursing home and home health agency owned by the same organization, as well as those within the community.

At the second level, a multiple services organization that is trying to establish a continuum internally will have to change its management structure and operating procedures to accommodate system-oriented goals and objectives. More teams, committees, and matrix management will be necessary, with the concomitant need for managers to spend additional time on coordinating their activities. For example, performance evaluations that were formerly done by a single supervisor may now require input from managers of several units. Strategic planning that focused on a single service must expand to consider the interaction of multiple services. When Lutheran General HealthSystem, now part of Advocate Health Care, decided to create the Continuum of Care for Chicagoland, they created 13 interdisciplinary task forces to address management issues ranging from extended care pathways to marketing.

The third structure level considers the relationships between separate organizations that agree to collaborate to provide a continuum. More than just patient transfer agreements, participation in a continuum implies acceptance of joint responsibility for the patient for the duration of his or her illness and extending to his or her well-being. For example, a nursing home that contracted with a hospital to provide its subacute care found that it had to incorporate hospital staff into its patient care conferences, introduce the role of the case manager from the hospital to the nursing home staff, modify patient records, coordinate patient education with hospital staff, and make other changes in its standard operating procedures—changes far beyond modifying its clinical procedures to accommodate a different type of patient. Similarly, the hospital arranged for its staff to participate in patient care conferences, patient and family education, and discharge planning at the nursing home. Nursing management at the nursing home and at the hospital had to coordinate patient and staff processes on an ongoing basis, which had not occurred previously.

At all levels of an organization, responsibilities, authorities, and communication must be consistent with the newly articulated goals and objectives that are systems-oriented rather than individually service-oriented. Figure 5-1 shows an organization with multiple services within the same parent organization. A diagram of patient flow shows that the patient is served by providers having quite different levels of organizational authority. Not surprisingly, patients did not characterize their care as "seamless," nor did staff. When the system did an internal analysis of referrals, it found that more than half of all referrals for all types of services went outside the system. Figure 5-2 shows a continuum of services provided by a hospital that owns or affiliates with a broad array of services, from wellness to acute hospitalization to long-term nursing home care. In this structure, patient care is orchestrated by a case manager. Figure 5-3 shows a network model of several community organizations bonded together through formal contracts and informal affiliations. In the latter two models, patient care is provided by staff at much more parallel levels of authority and responsibility, and integrating mechanisms (care coordination, shared patient record data, and inter-entity planning and management) facilitate communication throughout all levels of the organization.

Each continuum will be structured according to the unique characteristics of the services involved. A Continuum of Care Executive Management Committee is composed of the heads of each of the participating entities (for example, the CEO of the hospital, the president of the medical group, the owner of the nursing home, and the director of the home health agency). These are the people who have the authority to commit their organizations (or persuade their boards for commitment) and are the ultimate decision makers for their services. They must all agree on each entity's participation in the continuum. This committee is the group that creates the vision, defines the goals and objectives, and monitors the results of implementation.

A second committee comprises representatives of each participating entity who are responsible for the day-to-day operations, both clinical and administrative. The committee is referred to subsequently as the Continuum of Care Planning and Management Committee. Those participating may be the hospital vice president for patient care, the nursing home director of nursing, the case management coordinator of the social service agency, and the administrator of the medical group. In small organizations, such as an adult day care center, the person who participates in the Executive Management Committee may also participate on the operating committee because the single individual has internal responsibility for operations as well as overall direction of the service

Figure 5-1. Patient Flow in a Noncontinuum

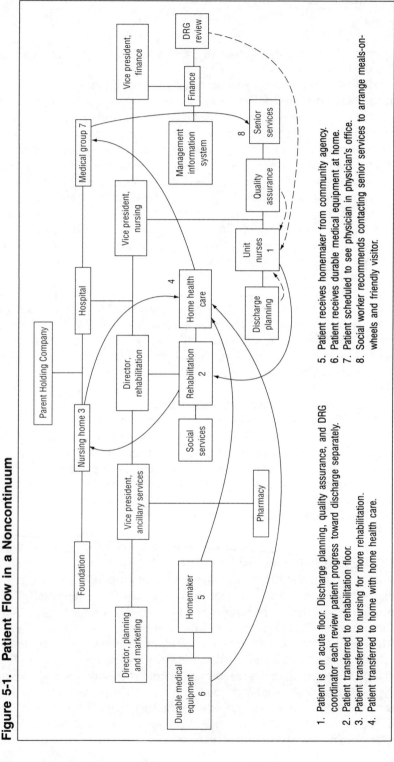

1. Patient is on acute floor. Discharge planning, quality assurance, and DRG coordinator each review patient progress toward discharge separately.
2. Patient transferred to rehabilitation floor.
3. Patient transferred to nursing for more rehabilitation.
4. Patient transferred to home with home health care.
5. Patient receives homemaker from community agency.
6. Patient receives durable medical equipment at home.
7. Patient scheduled to see physician in physician's office.
8. Social worker recommends contacting senior services to arrange meals-on-wheels and friendly visitor.

Source: Evashwick, C., and Weiss, L., editors. *Managing the Continuum of Care.* Gaithersburg, MD: Aspen, 1987. ©1987, Aspen Publishers, Inc. Reprinted with permission.

Figure 5-2. Example of Continuum of Care Organizational Structure, Hospital–Physician Model

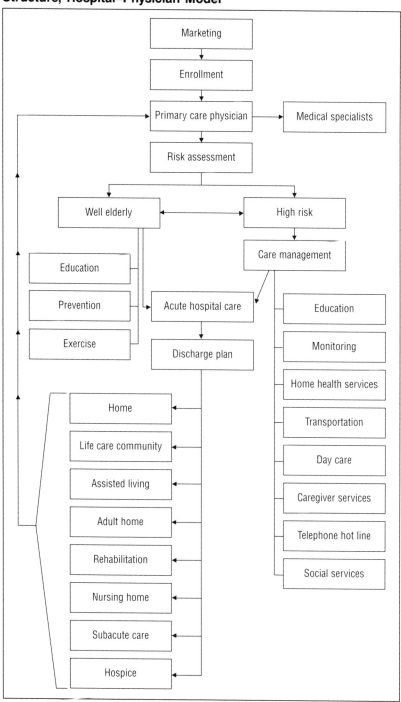

Source: Robert B. Scott, MD, Richmond Memorial Hospital, Richmond, VA, May 1996. Reprinted with permission.

Figure 5-3. Example of Continuum of Care Organizational Structure, Community Organization Network Model

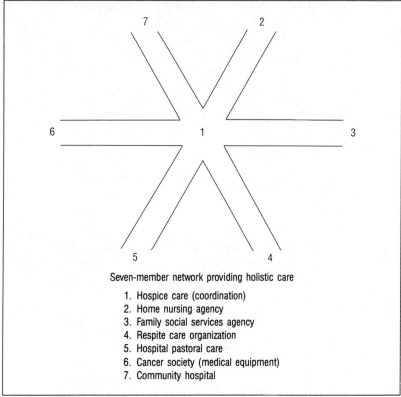

Seven-member network providing holistic care

1. Hospice care (coordination)
2. Home nursing agency
3. Family social services agency
4. Respite care organization
5. Hospital pastoral care
6. Cancer society (medical equipment)
7. Community hospital

Source: Adapted from Alter and Hage, 1993. Published in Evashwick, C. *The Continuum of Long-Term Care: An Integrated Approach.* Albany, NY: Delmar, 1995, p. 149. ©1996, Delmar Publishers. Reprinted with permission.

entity. This committee assumes responsibility for deciding collectively upon issues such as patient transfer procedures and for implementing the decision within their own organizations. This committee would meet regularly and would guide and assist the Director of the Continuum of Care, described below.

A single individual is designated as the Continuum of Care Director. This person has the vision to push continuum development to the next stage as well as the day-to-day responsibility for coordinating the activities of the participating entities. The Continuum of Care Director will probably not have direct authority for any clinical staff or administrative departments, but will have direct access to those in senior management positions. Tasks range from identifying the agenda for meetings of the Continuum of Care Executive Management Committee to convening a year-long task force to explore issues and initiate an integrated information system. If the continuum is primarily bringing together services within a single multi–health care system, the Continuum of Care Director should be situated fairly high within the corporate structure, have a budget and direct access to senior management, report to the president, and have delegated authorities. If the continuum is more of a network model, the position may be funded by a pooled budget and function more through influence and persuasion than direct authority. In either case, the Continuum of Care Director should work closely with both the Executive Management Committee, because it is the ultimate decision maker, as well as with the Continuum of Care Planning and Management Committee, because it has day-to-day responsibility for operations and immediate authority over staff.

As the continuum of care evolves, and organizations gradually change to system-orientation, the participating entities' belief in the continuum and ability to work together will strengthen. The Continuum of Care Director's direct authorities may also increase over time because, by definition, the continuum will always require coordination of numerous services, not all of which will be within a single corporate entity. The position of the Continuum of Care Director will always depend on influence, persuasion, and the ability to work convincingly with those who have direct-line authority.

Finally, short-term task forces and/or ongoing subcommittees may be convened to focus on specific issues. Task force and subcommittee members should include experts on the issues and represent some or all of the participating entities, as well as select individuals from the Continuum of Care Planning and Management Committee. Task forces may design an integrated information system or develop a standing committee to coordinate marketing efforts among the participating entities.

Following are the structure and management tasks discussed in this chapter:

- Start with each service.
- Establish the basic structure.
- Decide who should manage.
- Define tasks and responsibilities.
- Revamp management authorities.
- Expand clinical authorities.
- Implement inter-entity planning.

Start with Each Service

The concept of continuum of care used throughout this book implies coordination of many services beyond those available from a single participating entity (although a few very large multi–health care systems may indeed have a wide array of services). Before embarking upon formal relationships with external organizations, it is useful to examine the level of seamlessness inside. As figure 5-1 shows, internal patient flow can be chaos, particularly if an organization has recently expanded or merged. A Continuum of Care Task Force convened at one 250-bed community hospital found that, within the walls of the hospital alone, a patient could easily be asked to show his or her Medicare card 12 times during one inpatient admission.

Recommended Actions

- Examine internal services for ease and coordination of patient flow, including use of ancillary services and transfers among services.
- Identify internal structural changes required to streamline transitions within the organization, such as creating a smart card with basic patient data, or revise maps and signs to guide patients and families from one service location to another.
- Define internal goals and objectives and evaluation criteria and methodology for assessing each service's success in participating in the continuum of care.
- Establish a Continuum of Care Clinical Task Force comprising physicians, nurses, and other clinicians to streamline the provision and to optimize coordination of clinical activities.
- Assess the status of the patient record and work with information systems experts to plan and implement an integrated patient record that spans services.

Establish the Basic Structure

Continuums of care involving multiple organizations may take any of several basic structural models. *Single ownership* is often found in large multi–health care systems that have added services over the years. This also is likely to be a first step: The organization organizes the services it already owns and then expands to include others. *Joint ventures* are particularly common among services requiring heavy start-up capital or specialized expertise, such as senior housing or high-tech home infusion therapy agencies. *Affiliations* are common when services are quite distinct and the organization's history or culture has created strong but separate strengths, such as affiliations between hospitals and social service agencies.

Structural arrangements may have an overriding legal or contractual basis, but the legal status is much less relevant than the operating relationships. The key is how to provide patients easy access to the services they need when they need them. The structure will evolve as the continuum moves through the initial planning stages to implementation, on-going operation, and subsequent expansion.

Recommended Actions

- Identify the service entities that are potential participants in the continuum and meet with them to discuss possible collaboration.
- Convene a Continuum of Care Executive Management Committee.
- Articulate the continuum's vision, mission, goals, and objectives in such a way that the benefits to each of the participating entities are clear (see chapter 2).
- Secure board commitment (as described in chapter 2).
- Collectively go through the client mapping process described in chapter 3 and the service assessment process described in chapter 4.
- Examine the service array of each of the participating entities to identify those competencies that are core to the continuum and those activities that are neither essential nor pertinent to the continuum. Help each entity understand and agree on the parameters of its participation in the continuum.
- Jointly explore structural options, including getting expert opinions from lawyers and accountants on legal, regulatory, and financial considerations. Financial status and board structure also should be examined for their implications for formal structure.
- Determine and act on the best structure for the continuum of care for the present time.
- Explore options for purchase, start-up, or affiliation of missing services or services that do not meet criteria for availability, accessibility, or quality (discussed in chapter 4). Determine how the structural options for adding new services affect, or are affected by, the continuum's original structure.
- Develop a phased plan for integrating and incorporating services, including financial projections that will contribute essential information to make buy-or-affiliate decisions.
- Develop a business plan to be shared by all participating entities that will reiterate goals, strategic priorities, expected outcomes, the rationale for the continuum's structure and management, and the process for planning and implementing the continuum.
- Reaffirm board commitment.

Decide Who Should Manage

The discrete characteristics of different services must be recognized for both patient care and management purposes. One of the common mistakes made by hospitals in the vertical integration trend of the mid-1980s was for administrators to believe that they could manage anything, from travel agencies to senior housing. The continuum management structure of each participating entity must recognize that it is essential that the person(s) responsible for day-to-day administration be an expert in the management of that particular service. Moreover, the administrators of all the services must have enough breadth of perspective, if not direct experience, to appreciate each other's management requirements so that they can work together to construct management systems that respect the individuality of each service, but work toward the coordination inherent in the continuum.

Recommended Actions

- Identify internal experts in the administrative and clinical aspects of each service who can be called on for assistance in planning, implementing, and evaluating services.
- Convene a Continuum of Care Planning and Management Committee composed of individuals representing each participating entity who have authority to make decisions on behalf of that entity on issues pertaining to daily operations.
- Create a position for a Continuum of Care Director or vice president. If several entities are involved, they should agree on a single individual who will act, at minimum, as coordinator of activities and communications. The director will work closely with the operation management committee.
- Interview stakeholders within the participating entities, as well as externally, and ensure acceptance of the new management structure.

Define Tasks and Responsibilities

Whatever the formal structure for the organizational relationship, in addition to each participating entity, every individual participant in the continuum should understand his or her new role (versus his or her traditional job within a more limited unit). New roles and responsibilities should be articulated, understood, and accepted. However, issues of "turf" should not be underestimated. The Eddy, now Northeast Healthcare, reported that its most effective means for creating "systems" thinking and collaboration among employees evolved out of picnics, softball games, and holiday parties convened on behalf of the continuum. These activities provided opportunities for staff at different entities to work together on tasks beneficial to all. With the help of individuals committed to the new system, people learned to overcome their fear of unknown processes and to work together instead of compete with each other.

Recommended Actions

- Engage staff in discussions about how functioning as part of a continuum changes their duties.
- Conduct formal meetings with counterparts/colleagues of other units of the continuum so that people get to know each other personally.
- Arrange informal opportunities for those participating in the entire continuum to get acquainted in informal settings.
- Write additions and revisions to existing job descriptions. Ask staff members to modify their own job descriptions as a way of helping each learn and accept his or her new role and responsibilities.
- Revise performance evaluation criteria and methods to reflect continuum tasks and new relationships.

Revamp Management Authorities

Operating as a collaborative continuum requires different authorities than managing a single service. Thus, management authorities need to be revamped to recognize control that may expand beyond former lines or that may extend to authority over staff employed by other units either within the same organization or in other participating entities. This is essentially matrix management. For example, the director of social services of a multi–health care system may once have supervised only the social workers of the hospital who functioned in inpatient settings. As the result of creating a continuum of care, he or she now may have authority over the social workers stationed in physicians' offices, nursing homes, or a freestanding cancer center. Lutheran General Health-System created 13 separate management committees. Each committee spent 12 to 24 months developing detailed tasks and responsibilities for staff at all levels to articulate how the new continuum would be operated and managed.

Recommended Actions

- Create a sub-task force of the Planning and Management Committee composed of the managers of continuum services and support services to work together to define new management authorities that may cross traditional organizational lines.

- Have managers of participating entities meet regularly (for example, monthly) to discuss and resolve management issues.
- Establish short-term task forces.

Expand Clinical Authorities

Clinical authorities also may change due to the continuum. Where traditional clinical roles once might have ended, now they might be extended to enable clinicians to follow patients in other settings. Or, the sharing of information might be expanded from beyond what exists in the written record to verbal exchange and ongoing communication with clinicians of different venues. For example, the geriatrician who evaluated an elderly patient as part of an interdisciplinary geriatric assessment team might be asked to become medical director for the home health agency of a continuum and to work with the geriatrician who is medical director of the nursing home used by that continuum. Both might interact with the case manager from the managed care entity who would have the official task of shepherding the patient through the continuum of care created by the collaboration among the managed care entity, the physicians' medical group, the hospital, the nursing home, and the home care agency.

Recommended Actions

- Organize a task force of those clinicians involved in the continuum participating entities to articulate issues of patient flow among services and to develop processes to streamline efficiencies and enhance communication.
- Expand any existing interdisciplinary assessment team at the core of a continuum based in a hospital or medical group to include home health, step-down unit, and community-based agency clinicians as part of a continuum of care clinical team that meets regularly to discuss specific patients and general procedure issues.
- Initiate a medical grand rounds for the continuum of care, bringing together clinicians from many services to discuss complicated or exemplary cases on a monthly basis.
- Rewrite job descriptions to accommodate new responsibilities, as needed.

Implement Inter-Entity Planning

A continuum of care is likely to continue to expand, adapt, and otherwise evolve. The entities involved in the continuum, whether within the same organization or from several organizations, should consider their collective as well as individual futures. In large organizations and those that are part of large systems, planning often occurs in isolation from patient/client operations. On the other hand, in small organizations, particularly those that have been in business for a long time and have a stable set of services and clients, little formal planning may occur at all. Public agencies may plan only year to year, in accordance with federal, state, and local budget allocations. Whatever the constraints, the entities participating in the continuum should be working together for their future, as well as current operations. Strategic planning should be done from the continuum perspective.

Recommended Actions

- Establish a task force including representatives from all the participating entities that is devoted specifically to planning.
- Monitor the strategic directions and specific plans of each participating entity to ensure that the continuum remains a priority for all involved.
- Identify data gathered by any individual entity that can be shared with all the continuum participants. Also, identify data that can be used by all but are gathered by none, and then pool resources to gather the essential data.
- Develop a strategic plan specifically for the continuum of care, focusing each component of the plan on the entire continuum rather than on individual services or separate integrating mechanisms.

Chapter 6

Human Resources

Human resources issues are unlikely to be at the top of the list when administrators are negotiating creation of a continuum. Yet it is the human element that can make or break the successful implementation and operation of a seamless system of care.

Human resources issues range from technical financial and regulatory issues such as pay scales and portability of benefits, to softer yet critical issues such as motivation and promotion of teamwork, to strict management issues such as performance evaluation criteria and parity. The type and extent of human resources issues depends on where the seamless continuum falls on the own-to-affiliate range and on organizational culture. The entities participating in the continuum must address human resources individually, and would benefit by collaborating and sharing in some of the techniques to induce change. Also, changes made by one organization to accommodate the continuum, such as a change in job titles or pay scales, should be made known to the other entities participating in the continuum and should be consistent with the overall continuum management structure. Overall, the people involved in each of the entities participating in the continuum of care should understand its worth to the people they serve, their organization, and their own individual careers and needs.

The human resources function varies considerably among organizations. Hospitals are likely to have separate departments and very formal processes in place. Community-based social service agencies, on the other hand, may operate with a very small staff and a large cadre of volunteers. In trying to address continuum of care issues, those responsible for human resources in each of the participating entities should come together to identify common issues and areas in which they can assist each other to facilitate implementation of the critical human dimension of continuum management.

Following are the human resources tasks discussed in this chapter:

- Motivate staff to accept change.
- Analyze and revise job descriptions.
- Engage in team building.
- Evaluate employee performance.
- Establish pay parity.
- Consider portability of benefits and vestiture.
- Work out issues of unionization.
- Examine staff-spanning services.

Motivate Staff to Accept Change

Moving from individual services to a continuum of care requires a shift in thinking, different tasks, a new way of interacting, time taken from already busy schedules, and perhaps adoption of a new culture. Staff must understand the what and why if they are to participate effectively. The basic principles of organizational change should be considered and incorporated into planning a continuum. Staff must be involved early on, educated about potential and portending change, empowered to participate in creating new systems, continually informed with updated communications, and rewarded for facilitating the evolution of the organization. The human resources staff should be involved from the moment the administrators embark on the process of creating a continuum so that the human dimension receives the attention required.

Recommended Actions

- Include on the task force planning the continuum or the ongoing managing committee representatives from the human resources staff of the participating entities.
- Incorporate time and a plan for educating staff about the continuum.
- Have the human resources department, or the individual responsible for human resources in each of the participating entities, develop a plan explicitly for motivating staff to change in the direction of the seamless continuum.
- Ask all staff for their suggestions on changes that would move the organization toward seamlessness.
- Create rewards for various contributions to the new directions (for example, continuum of care employee of the month, best liaison with community agencies, most collaborative team, and so on).

Analyze and Revise Job Descriptions

In changing orientation from an individual service approach to a continuum of care, job descriptions should be evaluated and revised. Tasks and responsibilities should reflect collaboration with multiple services and instill expectations of working within the new system. Questions on past experience should ask about involvement with a variety of services and integrating mechanisms. Abilities should include a predisposition for collaboration and teamwork. Job descriptions also should be consistent and complementary across the different services involved in the continuum. As it began to expand its continuum, Beverly Hospital, in Beverly, Massachusetts, found that each of the services it added had different job descriptions for the same title. For example, case management: "Case management coordinator" in the acute hospital was a registered nurse who ensured adherence to clinical guidelines for the few days a patient was in the hospital; in the home health agency, it was a nurse who organized community-based support services and followed the patient over time; in the adult day care program, it was a social worker who helped clients process eligibility papers for federal, state, and local funding. Thus, the job descriptions had to be revised not only to reflect the activities within each organization, but also to achieve consistency across the organizations and services participating in the continuum.

Recommended Actions

- Develop and implement a process to revise all job descriptions to be consistent with continuum of care responsibilities and evaluation criteria.
- Jointly work with organizations participating in the continuum to revise job descriptions for inter-agency consistency.
- Ask staff to revise their own job descriptions based on the goals of the continuum and how their jobs have changed.
- Evaluate cross-training opportunities and job exchange programs for managers, clinicians, and support staff to provide intercontinuum work experiences as a basis for redesigning job content.

Engage in Team Building

Most continuum activity, particularly among clinicians, involves coordination with staff from different departments and/or organizations. Administrative and patient care teams are inherent in continuum of care activities as a basic method of coordinating actions across sites, over time, and among multiple disciplines. Thus, new and close working relationships must be developed with colleagues with whom there previously may have been little interaction. In addition, time must be devoted to collaborative and collective activities. Teams also will evolve as new staff join the organization and as the organizational configuration expands to include new members. For example, Lutheran General HealthSystem set up 13 task forces to create the Continuum of Care for Chicagoland. Each included staff from several provider entities. For the teams to be effective, administrators must allow time for and give sanction to planning, administrative, and clinical meetings. Shared goals must be developed, with measurable objectives, to evaluate and justify the continuation of the team. Someone must assume responsibility for setting up meetings, and attendees must be willing to travel off-site. Participating in teams is hard work; performance evaluations must be modified to reward positive participation in team efforts.

Recommended Actions

- Establish clinical teams to implement clinical coordination among the participating entities.
- Apply team-building principles to the task force convened to plan and implement the continuum.
- Allow time in the staff's schedules for team meetings.
- Engage in team-building exercises and team development, possibly engaging an outside consultant to conduct relevant activities.
- Set team goals and objectives or performance expectations so that meetings are productive and team members feel good about using their time for collaborative activities.
- Design ways for teams to evolve as new members join.
- Adapt continuous quality improvement (CQI) team-building principles and skills as applicable.

Evaluate Employee Performance

Most organizations evaluate employee performance on a regular basis using criteria that typically reflect an insular set of activities. However, as the continuum is developed, employees are asked to collaborate, interact across services, and "think" with a systems orientation. Thus, employee evaluation criteria should be changed to reflect these expectations; otherwise, employees will feel that they are not rewarded for participating in the continuum and may be reluctant to take the time or risks required for continuum activity. The new criteria should measure system-oriented activities and the employee's individual contribution to team efforts.

For example, the social workers responsible for discharge planning and service arrangement in a southern California hospital were evaluated on the number of referrals they made and how quickly they made them. When the hospital purchased additional facilities and services, no changes were made in the social workers' job descriptions or evaluation criteria. They continued with their previous patterns. The quickest path for referrals was to organizations with which they had already established relationships. A subsequent study by the hospital system revealed that more than 50 percent of all referrals for services were going outside the system to competitor home health agencies, rehabilitation providers, and durable medical equipment (DME) companies, despite the fact that the system now owned all these services. Only by changing the social workers' evaluation criteria and creating a new incentive structure was the hospital system able to redirect referrals internally.

Recommended Actions

- Develop new employee performance evaluation criteria to include continuum of care activities.
- Obtain employee input in articulating the challenges to acting as part of a continuum rather than as an independent service, and the activities that staff believe should be rewarded.
- Reward staff for continuum-oriented activities short term, as well as incorporating long-term measures into ongoing performance evaluation. For example, recognize a "Continuum of Care Initiative" employee or team of the month for the first 12 months of continuum development.
- Formulate a mechanism for incorporating the input of representatives from other participating entities in performance evaluations to allow the opportunity to recognize staff for positive interactions outside their own units.

Establish Pay Parity

Once services are all part of the same continuum, should all staff receive the same wages? Registered nurses, for example, have different pay scales in hospitals, doctors' offices, nursing homes, and home health agencies. This issue may be constrained by external forces. For example, reimbursement for nursing home employees may be capped by the state. Also, hospital DRG (diagnosis-related group) rates take into account local wage scales. Nurses in private home health agencies may be paid per diem or per hour, with no fringes, whereas nurses working for a Medicare-certified home health agency are as likely to be on straight salary.

In the early 1990s, the Sisters of Mercy of Farmington Hills, MI, had separate corporations for its aging services and its hospitals. When Sisters of Mercy began the process of integrating the hospitals and nursing homes, it decided to increase the salaries of the nursing home nurses to the level of those of the hospital nurses, even though the formula for state reimbursement for nursing homes did not accommodate the increase. They also instituted a long-term plan to offer benefits to all employees of the nursing home. On the other hand, Fairview, in Minneapolis (see chapter 16), faced similar issues but decided to go in the opposite direction. In order for Fairview's skilled nursing facilities to remain competitive within the constraints of state payment levels, its long-term care affiliate, the Ebenezer Society, remained a separate 501(c)(3) corporation, with Fairview as its sole stockholder. In this way, the Ebenezer Society facilities were able to maintain separate pay scales from the hospital and physician components of the parent organization.

Recommended Actions

- Find out whether there are indeed differences in pay scales and benefits for similar positions in different services of the continuum. (This information may be difficult to secure if the organizations are collaborating or affiliating, but not in formal ownership or management agreements.)
- Calculate the financial implications for the continuum if pay scales and benefits were to be made similar.
- Survey the staff of all services to learn whether their perception is that differences in pay or benefits exist, and, if so, whether this perception creates a serious morale problem.
- Ask staff what benefits they value other than salary, including intangible rewards.
- Consider revising job descriptions instead of all pay scales.
- Make a conscious decision about the course of action to take and communicate it to employees.

Consider Portability of Benefits and Vestiture

If continuum services become part of the same parent corporation, are employees allowed to transfer from one subsidiary company to the other and keep their benefits? Can they become vested by counting the total years in the corporation? If a hospital that has one retirement plan joins with a medical group that has another, external constraints may make it difficult, if not impossible, for the health care system to merge its existing retirement programs. Thus, a new retirement program may have to be set up for future employees, and old plans maintained or transitioned out over time. This issue does not apply to affiliations or collaborative arrangements that do not involve ownership or merger. Nonetheless, because affiliations are often first steps to eventual merger, the issue should be examined.

Recommended Actions

- Bring together the individuals responsible for human resources for each of the participating entities to identify potential challenges to combined vestiture, portability, and retirement plans. Consider both legal constraints and corporate cultural preferences.
- Engage human resource consultants to propose solutions to complex problems.

Work Out Issues of Unionization

In recent years, unions have increased their efforts to target health care workers. When a service that is unionized merges with, or is purchased by, a service that is not unionized, union issues must be worked out. For example, depending on the respective number of employees in the two organizations and the details of their union contracts, a union election may have to be held. The union can be counted on to (1) not want to lose its current members, and (2) fight as hard as possible to recruit all the members of the other organization. For example, when a unionized nursing home in New York merged with a nonunionized hospital, the hospital was forced to raise the salaries of the nurses in its subacute unit, which then caused a domino effect of raising the salaries of all the hospital's nurses. The action had serious, unexpected financial ramifications for the hospital and caused it to regret ever having purchased the nursing home. Even affiliations give the union an opportunity to reach new employee groups, so organizations collaborating in network models of the continuum also should be aware of the union status of their potential partners.

Recommended Actions

- Find out if any of the potential participating organizations are unionized.
- If a merger or purchase is impending, have a labor lawyer and human resources expert evaluate the potential financial and legal implications of the action before the terms are finalized. Alternative organizational and legal structures may be warranted.

- Educate employees about the pros and cons of unionization before the union has the opportunity to do so.

Examine Staff-Spanning Services

It sounds ideal to have staff who can follow patients through the continuum. For example, the physical therapist would work with the patient on the medical–surgical unit, in the skilled nursing unit, at home through home health, and later in the outpatient clinic. In the process of creating hospital joint ventures for home health, the LHS system in Los Angeles considered having staff who would go from inpatient hospital rehabilitation units to homes only to find that, in practice, it did not work out. Staff tend to self-select the type of setting in which they prefer to work. For example, home health agency staff tend to like flexibility of schedule and independence, just as emergency department staff enjoy the intensity of acute needs and teamwork. Given the diversity of settings comprising the continuum, not all staff will want to work in all settings. Moreover, rarely are all services provided under the same corporate umbrella, which means staff have different bosses, different salary structures, and a need to use different regulations governing reporting criteria. Finally, even if all the other details could be worked out, scheduling staff to span the continuum is problematic and does not guarantee that they would be on the service at the time the patient needed it. On the other hand, cross-training has become popular, at least within the context of the acute care hospital. In brief, the opportunities and problems with staff-spanning services should be evaluated carefully.

Recommended Actions

- Conduct a focus group of any staff who might be interested in working across services to ascertain whether spanning multiple services would be logistically possible and desirable from the staff's perspective.
- Interview staff who have worked in more than one setting, either simultaneously or sequentially, to learn the pros and cons of this working in several settings.
- Differentiate practical problems of staff-spanning services from human issues and deal with each separately.
- Delineate skill or knowledge differences that may accompany the same job in different venues.

Chapter 7

Case Management

Given the array of services included in the continuum, it is necessary to have some way of coordinating patient care. Care coordination is the second of the four integrating mechanisms defined in chapter 2 as essential to a continuum of care. This may be accomplished by any or a combination of several methods, including an individual designated as a case manager, an interdisciplinary team, or a clinical protocol. This chapter focuses on the issues of care coordination done as a separate function by an individual designated as a case manager. Chapter 8 addresses other means of care coordination.

Case management is a five-step process to assist patients who need complex and/or ongoing care and consists of case identification, assessment, care planning, service arrangement/implementation, and monitoring and reassessment.[1] Case management evolved from the role of the case worker in public government departments (social services, mental health, and public health nursing). During the 1970s and 1980s, national attention (and federal and state moneys) was given to demonstration projects in an effort to understand the role, cost, and value of case management. During the 1990s, case management has gained acceptance as a method for coordinating care across settings and over time. Care coordination is required by, or helpful to, many people with acute or chronic illness. However, case management is most cost-effective when targeted at patients with complex conditions requiring a range of services, with the possibility of changes in service, over a prolonged period of time.

In brief, a case manager assumes responsibility for a client/patient whose care plan may involve several different organizations, disciplines, or payers. He or she ascertains the need for services through either direct assessment or information received from other professionals, contacts service providers to arrange services, negotiates with payers (if necessary), and follows up with the patient to see if services have indeed been rendered and if additional or different services are needed. The case manager may or may not have formal authority to order services and/or authorize payment for services.

In the 1990s, case managers are employed by a full range of health-related organizations: hospitals, medical groups, managed care entities, home health agencies, community-based social service agencies, and health plans. Their responsibilities may vary. For example, their role may be condensed into a five-day hospital stay in the case of a nurse case manager orchestrating a hospital experience, or expanded to an ongoing monitoring role by a case manager based in a community social service agency. Case management is not yet a discrete job that requires a license, but certification is on the horizon. Several private organizations currently are advocating for certification and performance measured by quality standards. Certification may further define the case management function.

Funding for case management varies. Some states pay for case management through Medicaid waivers. Medicare pays for a limited amount of case management for select homebound patients through Medicare Part A for certified home health agencies. Some managed care companies and medical groups self-fund case management as an integral part of internal operations. In general, however, case management is not a reimbursable service covered by private health care insurance. (See table 7-1 for a summary of key characteristics of different types of case management.)

Following are the case management tasks discussed in this chapter:

- Delineate case manager authorities.
- Select case managers from the appropriate disciplines.
- Structure to support authority.
- Target appropriate clients.
- Set up case management mechanics.
- Cover case management costs.
- Coordinate multiple case management programs.

Delineate Case Manager Authorities

The authorities of case managers range from information and advocacy to full control over arranging services and guaranteeing payment. Each organization must decide the extent of its case managers' authorities. In medical groups and hospitals, where physicians and other clinicians are readily available, the case manager's decision-making autonomy may be less than in social service agencies or other settings where input or direction from clinicians is more difficult to obtain or not required by payers. In some instances, case managers may initially pose a threat to

Table 7-1. Summary of Key Characteristics of Case Management

Type	Population	Setting	Focus	Financing
Medical				
Primary care	Patients	Physician offices, clinics	Prevent, diagnose, treat, monitor	Private pay; Medicare; Medicaid; private insurance
Acute care	Patients	Hospital acute and subacute facilities	Facilitate flow of care, discharge, prevent readmission	Private pay; private insurance; Medicare; Medicaid
Other medical	Medically dependent; complex problems	Skilled nursing facility; home or special facility	Treat, monitor, supervise, prevent, rehabilitation	Private pay; private insurance; Medicare; Medicaid
Private insurance/ managed care	Enrollees; high risk; high cost	Private and acute settings	Authorize, verify services and utilization; manage benefits and costs	Private pay; private insurance; Medicare; Medicaid
Nonmedical				
Community/ in-home	Community-based; functional and cognitive disability	Noninstitutionalized	Coordinate wide range of nonmedical care; keep independent	Private pay; waiver funds; grants and contracts
Long-term care	Ongoing need for care or supervision; chronic problems	Community, in-home or facility	Monitor, prevent decline; link to needed resources	Private pay; private insurance; waiver funds
Mental health	Complex, chronic; psychiatric problems	In-home; community-based; group home	Education; life skills; adaptation compliance; monitoring	Private pay; private insurance; Medicaid; Medicare; grants and contracts
Other	Advice and counseling to the well	Community	Resource and service information; referrals	Private pay; grants and contracts

Source: White, M., and Gundrum, G. Case management. In: C. Evashwick, editor. *The Continuum of Long-Term Care: An Integrated Approach.* Albany, NY: Delmar, 1995, pp. 162–78. © 1996, Delmar Publishers. Reprinted with permission.

others, such as nurses, social workers, discharge planners, and utilization reviewers. For the case manager to be accepted as an integral and valuable part of the patient care team, his or her functions must be differentiated from those of existing professionals. This makes it easier for everyone to understand and accept the case management function. Clearly defining the case manager's role at the outset also circumvents the potential problem of the new case manager stepping beyond the role the organization has in mind.

Recommended Actions

- Define the goals of case management and make sure the position has sufficient authorities to accomplish them.
- Write a job description for the case manager that distinguishes that function from nursing, social work, discharge planning, utilization review, and other roles that might potentially overlap. This may also require rewriting the job description of other positions to avoid any potential for role duplication.
- Hire as the initial case managers people who have the knowledge to perform the task, but who also are known and liked within the organization and are politically astute enough to establish the role in a positive way.
- Document and publicize early success stories of patients and families helped by case management to use in educating physicians, staff, and new patients about its unique qualities and benefits.

Select Case Managers from the Appropriate Disciplines

Case management is a function and not a discipline-specific task. Case management can be done effectively by a nurse, a social worker, or a nonclinical person trained specifically as a case manager. Physical therapists, occupational therapists, and mental health counselors may serve as case managers for particular types of patients. Case management also may be the responsibility of a team, with the most appropriate and/or available professional on the team assuming the function for each individual patient. Health care organizations have found that the case manager's professional background is less important than his or her style, personality, ease at networking, and ability to overlook boundaries in preference for providing comprehensive care.

In a recent grant project funded by the Hartford Foundation to place case managers in physicians' offices, six sites around the country participated. Some of them used nurses, some used social workers, some used a combination, and others formed a team that included physicians. Health care organizations may employ case managers of different backgrounds in different parts of the organization due to subtle differences in function. For example, a social worker may be more effective in the geriatrics department helping seniors coordinate care in the community, whereas a registered nurse may be more effective helping cancer patients monitor home infusion therapy because their needs are likely to be more clinical. In general, nurses are likely to be more effective and/or better accepted in case management roles that involve frequent or intense clinical decisions. Similarly, social workers are likely to be more effective in situations involving extensive coordination of community-based services and determination of patient eligibility for public funding.

Recommended Actions

- Determine the knowledge base and skills required by the case manager. If these are discipline specific, note which discipline has the most appropriate training for the requisite expertise.
- Assess market availability of each potential discipline to determine if there are enough people with the desired training available in the local job market and if their salary is affordable.
- Consider historical relationships among professionals within the organization and in the community.
- Structure the case management program within the continuum so that, whatever their expertise, the case managers have access to those in other disciplines with complementary expertise.
- Allow the case managers to meet with those in other disciplines so that they can broaden their base of knowledge.
- Educate staff throughout the participating entities on the case manager role; assuage potential turf issues.
- As the initial case managers, choose people with knowledge of the organization and community, winning personalities, and expertise. First impressions count, and it is important that the first case managers demonstrate the value of the position and show how it complements, rather than competes with, other positions.

Structure to Support Authority

Where should case management be housed within the organization? Hospitals, physician practices, managed care entities, and social service agencies have displayed a wide range of management structures in which to house case management. Almost every permutation imaginable exists: social work case managers reporting to vice presidents for nursing services;

nurse case managers being part of discharge planning and reporting to social services; geriatric case managers reporting to the physician director of a geriatric assessment clinic; managed care case managers reporting to a nonclinical unit called Customer Services. In brief, there is no "one best way" to structure case management. The appropriate structure is determined by a combination of factors: the position's authorities, the patients targeted, and whether the function is for services within the institution or in the community.

In the 1980s and early 1990s, Huntington Memorial Hospital in Pasadena, CA, ran several case management programs simultaneously. An inpatient case management program, staffed by nurses, helped guide clients through their inpatient experience. The nurses reported to the director of nursing. Discharge planning in the hospital was staffed by social workers and worked closely with the case manager nurses, but reported to discharge planning, which ultimately reported to the vice president of patient services. A set of four case management programs funded by different sources helped patients obtain support services in the community. These case managers were social workers and reported to the director of the senior services program, who also reported ultimately to the vice president of patient services. The nurses and social workers of all the programs knew each other personally and shared information among themselves informally whenever the need arose.

Recommended Actions

- Reiterate the goals and measurable objectives of the case management function as it pertains to each participating entity and the continuum overall.
- Position case managers within each participating entity so that they have authority to accomplish their job.
- Articulate the role and authorities of the case manager in spanning across the participating entities so that inter-entity care coordination can be achieved as desired.
- Create formal structures and informal opportunities for case managers performing similar functions in different parts of the organization and in different participating entities to interact.

Target Appropriate Clients

Case management has been documented to be most cost-effective when targeted at high-risk patients who consume large amounts of resources and whose care may be streamlined with the assistance of case management support. It also has been found to be expensive and to generate additional service costs if used intensely for everyone, with no boundaries of service availability or appropriate targeting. In brief, to be cost-effective, case management must focus on specific high-cost, complex populations and services. The goals of the program must be consistent with the needs and patient care experiences of the target population selected. In its initial decisions about creating a continuum of care, an organization may have already focused on a particular target population – for example, high-risk mothers, older people with diabetes, young patients with spinal cord injuries. (See chapter 3.) *All* patients might thus be eligible for or automatically receive case management. However, if the target population is more broadly defined – for example, all seniors – case management may not be warranted for everyone. Explicit criteria for identifying patients to receive case management must be specified.

Recommended Actions

- Define the purpose of case management, the relevant target population, and the service parameters of the continuum.
- Identify the high-risk population for which case management has the potential to coordinate and streamline care.
- Establish explicit criteria for selecting patients/clients to receive case management and a process for assigning case managers to patients.
- Incorporate in evaluation criteria the data that can be used to measure case management's cost–benefit.
- If case managers perform multiple functions in addition to case management, establish a way of differentiating case management activities from other activities.

Set Up Case Management Mechanics

Setting up case management mechanics involves developing intake and referral forms, determining caseload size, creating a tracking system, setting criteria for client termination, and constructing an array of other operating procedures. Many organizations start with just one or two case managers. The function is new; a great deal of effort should be spent on role definition and the activities needed to gain acceptance by the organization's professionals and its affiliates. A great deal of time does not need to be spent reinventing all the mechanics of a case management program. At this point in the evolution of case management in the U.S., a proliferation of prototype programs exists, replete with forms, computer programs, job descriptions, and task analyses. These can be used as a basis and modified according to the unique needs of the continuum.

Recommended Actions

- Determine the basic model of case management to be used within the continuum.
- If any of the entities participating in the continuum has a case management function, draw upon their experience for tips in setting up the case management function for the continuum.
- Contact half a dozen similar organizations already using case management to ask their advice in program development.
- Attend one or more of the national conferences specifically on case management or that have a track on case management.
- Seek consultation from an expert to develop the mechanics for the program.

Cover the Costs of Case Management

As noted above, case management is not paid for by most third-party insurers as a direct patient care benefit. In reality, there are a variety of funding sources, including payers and provider entities themselves. For example, public programs that pay for case management for eligible patients include Medicaid and the Older Americans Act (OAA)/Area Agencies on Aging. The OAA and Medicaid, under waiver authorities, pay for case management programs that are then made available to those who are eligible under state or local entitlement regulations. Many managed care entities have their own internal case management programs, with full-time professional staff who serve as case managers to high-risk enrollees. Hospitals have created case management programs primarily for inpatient case management and paid for them with internal operating funds. And a number of case management programs have been initiated with grant funding, with the cost–benefit and ongoing funding determined over time. Good examples are the physician office practice models funded by the Hartford Foundation and the St. Mary Medical Center community-oriented case management program in Tucson, AZ.

Recommended Actions

- Determine the cost of case management, including staff salary and benefits, office space, and other indirect expenses.
- Place a cost value on the expected benefits of case management, as measured by the specified goals and objectives.
- Explore available funding sources such as public programs, private programs, grant initiatives, and foundation support.
- Give a start-up program two years to demonstrate that its benefit to the organization warrants the cost; revise the program according to its financial viability.

Coordinate Multiple Case Management Programs

In recent years, the need to coordinate patient care and the cost efficiencies to be gained by doing so have resulted in a proliferation of case management programs. Today, we are in the ironic situation of needing to coordinate care coordinators! One medical group that recently started a case management program found that its case manager was trying to coordinate care for a hospitalized patient who also was being served by the hospital's case manager for inpatient care, a home health liaison who was arranging a variety of home care services, and a managed care case manager. Although all shared the same overall goal of getting the patient the most appropriate care as efficiently as possible, each had different authorities and different objectives. In a continuum of care created through affiliation of several distinct entities, multiple case management functions might exist even within the same continuum.

Recommended Actions

- Identify all case management functions that affect the continuum, both those internal to the continuum entities and those operated by nonparticipating organizations.
- For case management functions within the continuum, compare job descriptions, authorities, objectives, and operating procedures. Examine the opportunities for combining the different programs into a single case management department serving all the participants of the continuum. Alternatively, if separate departments are to be maintained, set up a committee or other opportunities for case managers to share information and develop ways to coordinate their efforts.
- In dealing with multiple external case management programs, be clear about what your case management function does, its authorities and limits. Meet with the case managers and their superiors to clarify who has precedence and under what conditions. Look for ways to share information that would expedite the efforts of all case managers (for example, basic patient admission/discharge data).

Reference

1. White, M. Case management. In: G. Maddox, editor. *Encyclopedia of Aging.* New York City: Springer, 1987.

Chapter 8

Other Types of Care Coordination

The goal of care coordination, or care management, is to get patients access to the services they need when they need them as efficiently as possible. Thus, care management benefits patients and their families by ensuring that the care they receive is tailored to their needs and by helping them negotiate the complex health care system. It also benefits providers, many of whom may be based in different locations or organizations, by enhancing communication and coordination among them. Case management benefits payers by maximizing resource use and by decreasing costs through increased efficiency. Each continuum will develop its own mechanisms for care coordination. Case management (discussed in chapter 7) is one. Several others are outlined below.

Following are the care coordination tasks discussed in this chapter:

- Develop extended care pathways.
- Establish interdisciplinary teams.
- Facilitate single access to care.
- Set up information and referral programs.

Develop Extended Care Pathways

Clinical pathways, guidelines, and protocols are now common in acute care settings; however, extended care pathways are relatively rare. Care guidelines specify what services are to be used in what time frame and under what conditions. Typically they are triggered by acute events. Extended care pathways span patient care beyond the hospital or physician's office to include pre- and post-acute services. Most extended care pathways existing today have been developed by hospitals but include discharge to nursing homes, home care, or adult day care. The National Chronic Care Consortium (NCCC) has developed a white paper explicating extended care pathways,[1] and several of its members, as well as other select institutions, have developed prototypes.[2] Extended care pathways institutionalize coordination and service transition that might otherwise be done on an individual patient basis by a case manager.

Recommended Actions

- Research extended care pathways through NCCC documents or by contacting NCCC members or others who have developed them.
- Monitor the experience of organizations using extended care pathways to see if the models and their realized benefits would apply to your continuum.
- In designing extended care pathways, include those representatives of the entities participating in the continuum that are appropriate for the patient diagnosis.
- Analyze case management practices to see if referrals and service coordination can be standardized enough to become formalized into a written pathway.

Establish Interdisciplinary Teams

Teams are a time-tested means of coordinating complex care involving multiple professionals. Inpatient rehabilitation units in hospitals and nursing homes typically function with an interdisciplinary team composed of physicians, nurses, physical therapists, occupational therapists, speech therapists, nutrition counselors, pharmacists, and social workers. The team conducts a multifaceted assessment when the patient first arrives, then formulates a patient care plan. One of its members may be designated to follow the patient and family to coordinate the provision of services by both the team members and other providers, including community-based support agencies. This type of team is triggered by an acute event requiring active rehabilitation.

A geriatric assessment team is an example of a team that may be asked to see an older person at any point in time, precipitated by crisis or not. The team is interdisciplinary and involves professionals from each of the key disciplines who specialize in geriatrics. The assessment team may make a one-time review of the older person's condition, recommend a plan of action for the family, and then conclude its involvement. In some models, the geriatric team functions as a consult service only; in others, the team internist becomes the patient's primary care physician and a case manager may be assigned to work with the patient and family on a regular basis, with the rest of the team called in as needed.

Interdisciplinary teams typically are found within a single organization, although models do exist of teams that consist of professionals based in different organizations. Interdisciplinary teams are expensive to operate, and their services usually cannot be fully reimbursed. They are most cost-effective for patients requiring multiple clinical services on an intense and simultaneous basis.

Recommended Actions

- Evaluate the value of an interdisciplinary team to the identified target population.
- Calculate the volume of demand for use of the team to determine its cost-effectiveness.
- Analyze the costs of operating a team and explore current reimbursement sources, levels, and authorization requirements.
- Determine whether the expertise required for an interdisciplinary team is available within a single organization or within multiple entities participating in the continuum.

Facilitate Single Access to Care

A continuum having many services that predate its creation may find that patients and families enter the system from as many entry points as there are services. Although this may be a fact of history, it may become counterproductive to meeting patient needs when the continuum is fully operational. A single access system may actually increase referrals to the participating entities and enhance coordination of patient care. One organization that had most of the continuum services within a single parent corporation found that it had 10 different offices, with 10 different telephone numbers, and 10 different points of admission to its continuum. The organization concluded that it would be able to diagnose patient needs and arrange the appropriate services more efficiently if all call-in patients used a central number and if one central location scheduled first-time appointments.

In the case of a continuum serving AIDS patients, there were eight community organizations, each of which maintained completely separate organizations. To facilitate access, they agreed to establish a single phone line and to have all initial client assessments done by an interdisciplinary team based in one of the participating organizations. Patients received a central record and a defined care plan, and then were referred to the appropriate provider for ongoing care.

Single access may include telephone access, physical location access, triage, initial assessment, case management locus, and a locus for or source of central patient records.

Recommended Actions

- Once the participating entities of the continuum are in place, identify problems that occur because of multiple-entry sites and opportunities that could be gained by having a single access.
- Evaluate the practical problems involved in creating single access (for example, telephone lines in different area codes, geographic proximity).
- Conduct a focus group of patients to obtain their responses to multiple- and single-entry organizations.
- Work with the task force or individuals responsible for marketing the continuum to maximize communication with professionals and consumers so that whichever model is used, they know how to access the services they need when they need them.

Set Up Information and Referral Programs

Information and referral (I & R) programs are common in some sectors of the continuum of care, such as senior services, particularly those sectors sponsored by the Area Agencies on Aging. Usually, such programs provide a listing of services available, times, locations, and eligibility criteria, typically in a directory or computerized format. I & R programs and their variations are a means of facilitating communication about continuum services and may provide limited in-person assistance as well.

In the early 1990s, the Hartford Foundation funded a demonstration project to link physicians with the continuum of community-based services. Sites across the nation experimented with placing social workers or geriatric nurses in physicians' offices. Their function was not to provide clinical service but, rather, to assist patients and families in identifying resources within the continuum and elsewhere in the community that could meet their needs. The social workers and nurses also provided education and resource materials to the staff of the physicians' offices. The underlying concept was to develop a current catalogue of the full array of services offered by the entities participating in the continuum, as well as of other services in the community that might be needed by ill or well patients and their families, and to have an experienced professional available to assist patients and families in identifying needs and arranging resources, with feedback provided to the physician.

Many continuums of care, even those based primarily in one corporate entity, find that clinicians and support staff throughout the continuum are not always aware of the many services available, let alone how to access them. Whether made available to patients and families or to external community agencies, or used exclusively by the providers in the continuum's participating entities, a detailed directory of services would be helpful in facilitating patient access and provider coordination within the continuum.

Recommended Actions

- Delineate all the services available throughout the continuum, describe how to access them, and communicate this information to the clinicians, administrators, and support staff of participating entities.
- Update the directory regularly.
- Delineate additional resources available in the community.
- Seek existing listings of community resources and expand them to include all entities participating in the continuum of care.
- Set up an I & R program specifically for the continuum.
- Explore the financial and practical feasibility of having a skilled professional available to continuum clinicians to assist them in identifying and arranging for resources.
- Review job descriptions and activities of social workers and case managers throughout the continuum to see how an I & R function may complement or compete with their job. If the function already exists within the continuum, find a way to make it widely available.

References

1. National Chronic Care Consortium. *Conceptualizing, Implementing, and Evaluating Extended Care Pathways.* Bloomington, MN: NCCC, 1995.

2. NCCC. *Conceptualizing, Implementing, and Evaluating Extended Care Pathways.* Section 4: case studies of extended care pathways in two chronic care networks, pp. 40–51. Bloomington, MN: NCCC, 1995.

Chapter 9

Information Systems

Truly seamless care depends on the efficient and complete transmission of patient information. The ideal management information system (MIS) would fully integrate demographic, financial, clinical, and utilization data, from all care settings, in ways that could be used for clinical and management decision making. It would be computerized, and more than a fancy e-mail system or a common data repository, and the system would be interactive and available 24 hours a day by any authorized user from any substation. The system would eliminate information duplication, inconsistencies, and incompleteness.

At the present time, each service of the continuum operates its own data system. Moreover, the clinical, financial, and management data systems within each service are likely to be separate. Although we are being driven to believe that the information highway is taking over, paper records are still the norm for clinical data. These are further split into physician orders, nursing notes, lab reports, X-ray results, prescriptions, and notes from other providers. Thus, if a patient sees multiple physicians and uses several pharmacies, comprehensive information on that patient may not be stored anywhere. Many social service and other community-based agencies still maintain key patient information on 3 × 5 cards in a manual system. The fragmentation of records is further complicated by the fact that the content and format of information gathered by a particular provider may be specified by state and/or federal mandate.

Like service providers, payers do not have complete patient records. Insurance companies may maintain utilization data, but only for the services they cover. With managed care a driving force for service integration, providers are trying to integrate clinical data with utilization and financial data in order to calculate an accurate capitated rate, adjusted for the clinical condition of either the individual or a specific patient population. But as providers assume risk, health plans may require fewer data. Thus, if a patient switches providers or uses providers outside the provider network, neither payer nor provider may have a complete record of the patient's service use. Except for Medicaid, most major payers do not cover long-term care, so nursing home, home health, and other long-term services provided over an extended period of time are not likely to appear in records maintained by acute providers.

Although prototypes are feasible and in process, no comprehensive turnkey commercial product that fully integrates clinical, financial, and management data for acute and long-term care services across different service settings yet exists. The overall expense has been reduced due to technical advancements, but computer and personnel costs remain high, and the benefits of comprehensive information systems in terms of cost reduction and quality enhancement have not yet been proven. Regardless, payment mechanisms and quality measurement will force the integration of data systems.

St. Mary Medical Center in Long Beach, California, typifies a community hospital at the forefront of installing a comprehensive, computerized MIS. The center is working department by department to implement computerized patient care records, including the capability of delineating clinical guidelines within the record. For example, the obstetrics clinic and the delivery room, each of which has its own records, will be mutually accessible. The laboratory and X-ray departments are already computerized. An interface engine is being installed to enable lab and X ray to be accessed on-line—real time—with the patient's inpatient and outpatient records. Physicians' offices, both on- and off-campus, also are connected. Home health, which has its own information system, also will be linked, although some software adaptations will be required to translate patient identification numbers.

The hardware capability exists to link the IPA (independent practice association) management company and the major health plan(s) with which the physicians and hospital contract. Pharmacy data, which are maintained by the health plans, and required authorizations, done by the IPA, will be able to be incorporated into the system and, as with the other components, accessed by the physicians on-line, in real time. New software will be developed to link each of the additional components to the integrated patient record and to translate from the different databases without major changes in data collection by each of the participating entities. Community-based nursing homes and social service agencies will be given the opportunity to come on-line in the future.

The issues confronting organizations in developing an integrated MIS for the continuum include all the people, content, and mechanics issues faced when implementing a single information system, compounded by integrating several information systems simultaneously, and multiplied by an order of magnitude in dealing with several service providers. As mentioned earlier, a fully integrated, interactive computerized system is the ideal, and neither the complexity nor the costs of the ultimate product should be a deterrent to striving for the ideal. Each information system must begin with the people who will use it, articulating their data needs and creating a paper system that works as the framework for the ultimate MIS. The computerization mechanics then follow. The costs of hardware and software can be spread over time as the continuum evolves. Knowing the MIS desired for the future will direct decision making each time that an information system is purchased, expanded, or modified; having the long-term goal will help prevent further fragmentation of information systems.

Following are the information systems tasks discussed in this chapter:

- Involve the appropriate people.
- Articulate information needs.
- Ensure hardware conformity and capacity.
- Ensure software conformity and capacity.
- Link software.
- Establish common codes and format.
- Recognize and respect mandatory differences.
- Ensure security of and access to information.
- Control costs.
- Provide training for staff.

Involve the Appropriate People

Often information systems are the purview of computer gurus or financial experts. The system for the continuum of care should be developed by a multidisciplinary team composed of clinicians, administrators, and MIS experts. Such a task force may include a subset of the representatives on the continuum of care planning committee but should be expanded to include staff who deal with data in each of the participating entities. An appropriate system cannot be created without the content input of the people who will be using it. Physicians are particularly hard to convince about the value of learning and using new information systems. It is especially difficult to persuade older physicians of the virtues of computerized clinical records. Thus, if an MIS is to be used by physicians, it is essential that they be involved in its conceptualization and development. In addition, the computer field is moving so quickly on integration issues that current MIS expertise is absolutely essential. If no MIS expert is available from any of the participating components, a consultant should be engaged who has documented, recent experience creating the type of system at issue. Just as the continuum involves collaboration among many partners, so does the information system that will be used to manage it.

Recommended Actions

- Convene a data task force of clinicians and administrators representing the various services comprising the continuum, as well as staff experts representing finance/accounting, information systems, and quality assurance. (Consider including representative payers [health plans].)
- Involve physicians in data systems development and find a champion who will persuade colleagues of the system's value.
- Establish an ongoing committee of MIS staff responsible for the technical components of each entity's system to share developments, solve problems, and plan joint actions.
- Engage experts in information systems as consultants if necessary.
- Involve the human resources department or whatever unit(s) is responsible for in-house education to conduct frequent training sessions pertinent to the integrated MIS. Bring together staff from the various entities involved so that they can get to know each other and engage in collective problem solving, as well as learn the technical aspects of the system.

Articulate Information Needs

Consistent with the definition of a continuum of care, the goal of the MIS is to be able to guide and track patients over time through a comprehensive array of services and to include the clinical, financial, utilization, and management information necessary to achieve cost-effective patient care.

The first step in building such a system is to determine in detail what and how much information is needed by multiple providers or units. For example, St. Elizabeth Hospital in Lincoln, Nebraska, convened a Continuum of Care Information Systems focus group. In identifying representatives of departments who gathered data pertinent to patient flow just within the inpatient hospital, the administration identified 18 individual units. The 18 members of the focus group each brought lists of the data they collected. A comparison of the lists revealed multiple duplications, such as the eight separate units that asked for the Medicare number. The charge to the continuum of care committee then became to streamline data collecting. Likewise, the National Chronic Care Consortium (NCCC), which comprises 27 health networks with primary, acute, and long-term care institutions collaborating to develop continuums, formed a year-long task force to develop data elements common to the various providers of the continuum. The task force gained consensus on a core data set applicable to acute and long-term care service providers.

Recommended Actions

- Convene an Information Systems Task Force to focus on the continuum's MIS needs.
- Collect the information currently being gathered by the various units of each participating entity (for example, examples of admissions forms, discharge forms, billing and patient records).
- Determine a basic core of data useful to, or required by, multiple units.
- Identify data that are collected but not needed by anyone and delete.
- Test the usefulness of data gathered by one unit to another unit, within the same or different entities, by sharing paper or computer records on a sample of cases.
- Track several patients who use multiple services to see what happens to their records as they move from one provider to another.
- Formulate a plan for streamlining information collection, incorporating the sharing of information by paper or computer methods.
- Identify, in advance, the joint reports that all the continuum participants would like to receive.
- Think ahead to measuring quality and performance evaluation, identifying those measures that should be incorporated into the information system.

Ensure Hardware Conformity and Capacity

In the 1980s, having hardware at all, let alone compatible hardware, was a major issue. Today, most organizations have computers and software translation programs that make it fairly easy to go across platforms. But even so, trying to link all services of the continuum with a shared information system may reveal that some have computers that are out of date and/or require upgrading in order to be able to process either the volumes of potentially available information or the software required for linkages. And even though new operating platforms and translation programs facilitate communication, switching between operating systems may be problematic. Finally, social service and housing entities may still have only minimal computer systems or none at all.

Recommended Actions

- Assess each participating entity's hardware configuration, including operating platform, capacity, and linking capability.
- Determine how external communications are done: by modem, through a data line, a telephone line, by fax, or through the Internet.

- Develop consensus about hardware type and minimal requirements.
- Determine requirements and options for linking.
- Calculate the budget requirements needed to get every station to minimum capability over a defined period of time (such as 5 years).
- Set up a time frame for hardware and software purchases consistent with the budget of each participating entity.
- Explore discounts for hardware purchases in quantity.

Ensure Software Conformity and Capacity

Advances in software and translation programs make it possible for computer systems that once were totally incompatible now to be linked together or to have information translated easily from one system to another. Increasingly, software is written with open architecture that is designed from the start to interface with other software programs. Nonetheless, the varying levels of sophistication and currency of the MISs of the entities participating in the continuum may pose a challenge for the immediate sharing of information, and systems translation is frequently not as simple as it is supposed to be.

Recommended Actions

- Inventory the software available at each provider site, including clinical, financial, and management software. Note both the type of program (word processing, spreadsheet, graphics) and version. Make special note of linking programs.
- Determine the potential of each software program to communicate with similar programs (for example, can all word-processing programs be translated into one another; can database programs be translated into other database programs) and to be interfaced with other programs (can the word-processing program be used with the graphics program).
- Explore discounts for software purchased in quantity or for multisite use.
- Develop a plan for acquiring common software over time.

Link Software

Organizations that have recognized the need for integrated information have discovered that there is no existing software program that does everything the ideal system should. Thus, a number of organizations have embarked on creating their own software. For example, the former

Lutheran General HealthSystem (now Advocate) in Park Ridge, Illinois, committed $25 million over a five-year period to develop its software. The UniHealth America system in southern California has embarked on a multiyear software development initiative at a cost of more than $40 million. However, for the average community hospital, small medical group, or community-based agency, these sums are unrealistic and not necessary. The good news is that software vendors are aware of the increasing demand for integrated systems and are in the process of developing prototypes. Similarly, those large systems that are developing software will have products within the next several years, and some may be in a position to sell them. Fully integrated data systems are the long-term goal. In the interim, linking specific services and/or specific components of records are ways to begin, with full integration phased in over time as software evolves.

Recommended Actions

- Determine what software each service of the continuum is currently using.
- Determine what potential and options exist for linking existing software (for example, e-mail, Internet, LAN capability) and determine software and communication systems hardware requirements (data lines, telephone lines).
- Examine the software currently available for integrating discrete activities (for example, integrating admissions and scheduling).
- Formulate short- and long-term solutions for linking.

Establish Common Codes and Format

Organizations (and individuals) create their own ways of recording information. For example, the Information Systems focus group convened by St. Elizabeth, mentioned earlier, found that the same information was recorded in different ways within its own organization and thus could not be matched electronically across units. For example, some units recorded a name as First, Middle, Last, and some recorded it as Last, First, Middle. Some used the full middle name, and others used only the middle initial. Each unit also created its own identification number. The outpatient department gave each patient a unique number for each visit (making it impossible to track the aggregate experience of someone with a common name, let alone match inpatient to outpatient records). In some situations, recording practices were based on a specific rationale, or even regulated. Much of the time, however, routine practice was based on personal preference or history. Standardized ways of recording medical and health-related data have been developed and offer ready-made conformity if all of the entities participating in the continuum can agree upon which method to use.

Recommended Actions

- Identify the common information collected by multiple units.
- Develop a common core data set to be used by all participating entities.
- Determine (by consensus or mandate) common ways that the same information will be gathered by each entity. Make this method computer appropriate from the start, even if computerization will not take place until a later date.
- If data are to be shared immediately, create a translation code book that enables one entity to know how another entity has coded a particular item or where the information is located on the form or in the computer file.
- Phase in implementation of agreed-upon usage. (Allow time to use up all the existing forms in order to minimize the cost of change; use new recording formats on replacement forms.)
- Develop a code book that explains how various data are to be specified, making it as complete yet simple as possible, or adapt one of the existing coding systems.
- Evaluate compliance with uniform code usage over time and update as new data requirements emerge and new entities participate in the continuum.

Recognize and Respect Mandatory Differences

Some entities record information in ways that are essential to its function, but inconsistent with the way similar information is reported by other similar units. For example, hospitals record utilization in days, Medicare-certified home health agencies in visits, private home care in hours; obstetrics departments report activities as deliveries, and rehabilitation departments report activities as 15-minute increments of therapy. Starting and ending dates for fiscal years may vary for different participating entities of the continuum. In addition, core databases may differ: Managed care companies record enrollees, hospitals record short-term patients, physicians' offices maintain records of active and inactive patients, and senior centers may keep rosters of everyone who attended anything during the preceding year. Finally, state and federal requirements may affect data. For example, a nursing facility is required to gather minimum data sets (MDSs) on all patients, regardless of whatever other records it may have obtained from the hospital or physician's office. At one time, the Senior Care Network of Huntington Memorial Hospital in Pasadena, California, ran four separate case management programs, each having a separate and distinct computerized database. Three of these programs were state supported, and each had its own regulations and a state-mandated data set.

Recommended Actions

- Recognize differences in content and/or format that cannot be changed by the will of the participants in the continuum.
- Try to accommodate duplications or overlaps through software and/or code book adjustments.
- Identify the most elementary set of common information and focus initial collaboration on those elements for which consensus can be gained.
- Create a long-range plan for overcoming barriers to integration.
- Establish an ongoing information systems review as one function of the committee or management team overseeing the operations of the continuum.

Ensure Security of and Access to Information

Many of the issues that arise in creating an integrated information system are the same issues that occur in installing a new information system for a discrete function or task—they are simply magnified because of the multiple sites and services involved. Security is one example. Every patient care data system carries the potential threat of loss of patient confidentiality. This is compounded when multiple services, and possibly multiple organizations, are involved and when the patient's record is more comprehensive than ever before. The replies to those who express concern are: (1) Access can be limited to those with legitimate reasons for knowing the patient's identity, just as it can be for more discrete systems; and (2) the trade-off to the patient of having more information revealed should be enhanced quality.

Recommended Actions

- Develop a plan for information systems implementation similar to that which would be developed for a discrete system, allowing more time for staff training, problem solving, and testing.
- Make sure that help numbers are available at all times to all participating entities.

Control Costs

The costs of creating an integrated information system range from very little to the multimillion dollar efforts being undertaken by some of the large health care systems. The initial cost is the time of the staff involved to tackle the content and process issues outlined above. The more entities participating in a continuum, the greater the number of manpower hours that will be required. However, the initial input from users is essential to create a usable system. The earlier and more complete the process of delineating the core data system, developing common codes, and streamlining the data collection process, the more efficient and useful the information system is likely to be. The costs of additional software may be partially offset by incorporating changes pertinent to integration into software purchases that were already planned and budgeted. Moreover, if several organizations and/or service entities are acting collectively, their combined information system budgets may be enough to purchase the software required for integration and still meet the needs of the individual units. For example, a new pharmacy software program could be written or purchased with the hooks to link into the nursing software, the patient identification number could be specified to match, and minor programming could be done to accomplish the integration.

Many software programs currently are being advertised as "integrated." These must be evaluated carefully to determine whether a product that will meet the needs of the continuum exists or must be developed; the costs associated with each obviously vary.

Recommended Actions

- Determine the costs needed to purchase or upgrade the hardware needed for the desired information system. If several entities are participating in the continuum, explore discounts for volume purchases and ascertain whether any of the involved entities is part of a group-purchasing organization that could get a discount for all of the entities involved.
- Once the general parameters of the desired information system are articulated, explore existing software to see if any meets the needs.
- Consider pooling funds from the entities participating in the continuum to purchase or develop an information system that will serve all the entities.
- Take a long-term perspective in building the information system, spreading costs over several years.
- Incorporate systems-design requirements into information systems purchases that have already been budgeted.

- Offer to beta-test integrating software being developed by commercial companies.

Provide Training for Staff

All information systems require training of the staff who are to use the system at all levels—gathering data, inputting data, preparing reports, and using reports. Training for use of an integrated MIS is critical. This is a new level of information exchange and represents what may be, for many of the staff involved, a new concept in care giving. Many of those involved may be accustomed to only one component of data within their own entity. The new information system being designed and implemented will ideally integrate clinical, financial, and management information from within the organization, as well as data across all of the participating entities and over time. The new system's complexities must be carefully explained to users; otherwise, it will not be used to its full potential and, worse, may prove inaccurate or incomplete because data have not been gathered or entered accurately. Training for the information system offers the positive side benefit of providing an opportunity for those working in different participating entities to get to know each other within a shared problem-solving, educational context.

Recommended Actions

- Conduct training sessions for all staff of all entities and units involved with any aspect of the information system.
- Hold regular, ongoing training sessions to accommodate staff turnover.
- Identify physician and other clinical champions to help educate and persuade their colleagues of the benefits of the MIS.
- Provide feedback to staff on how the information system is being used and how its use could be improved or enhanced.
- Listen to staff complaints of difficulties with the information system and consider these in making refinements to the system.
- Experiment with having staff from one unit participate in teaching those from other units about the information system.

Chapter 10

Financing the Continuum

Financing is one of, if not *the,* most challenging aspects of constructing a seamless continuum of care. The current mechanisms for financing health care are highly fragmented and thus provide a major obstacle toward integration at any level. For example, the definition of continuum of care assumes that its goal is to integrate acute and long-term care services, yet insurance for acute care does not include long-term care, and insurance for long-term care does not include acute care. Medicare, which covers care for those age 65 and older, does not cover long-term care, despite the fact that most Medicare beneficiaries have chronic conditions. Medicaid covers many long-term care services but is limited to patients who have low incomes. An array of public and private social service programs pay for services that support those patients with acute or long-term care needs, but provision of and payment for services is entirely separate from other health care services. (See table 10-1 for current sources of funding for continuum services.)

Ideally, funding for the continuum of care would be capitated, with the service package tailored to meet the needs of each individual without the constraints of categorical funding. The capitated amount would include funds for acute care, long-term care, screening, prevention, diagnosis, and treatment. In other words, it would cover the full spectrum of services an individual would need over time. However, this approach would require combining financing for acute and chronic care and social support services (as well as perhaps housing). Such broad financing by third-party payers, private or public, does not reflect how health care financing in the U.S. has developed historically. Moreover, we do not have data at a national level that accurately tell us how much it costs to provide comprehensive, efficient care over time to people with chronic or long-term illnesses. Nor do we have universally accepted models that enable us to identify patterns of individuals who would be high or low users of services, or users of one type of service configuration or another. Without utilization data on which to base financing, and absent a philosophy that places no limits on service funding, funding for the continuum is likely to remain a challenge. Operating a continuum in the current environment requires a creative combination of existing financing mechanisms with less financing fragmentation.

Following are the financial management tasks discussed in this chapter:

- Maximize basic sources of funding.
- Explore secondary sources of funding.
- Negotiate with third-party payers.
- Implement case management.
- Initiate fund-raising.
- Monitor demonstrations.
- Advocate private responsibility.

Table 10-1. Sources of Funding for Services of the Continuum

Service Provider	Sources of Funding
Extended care (Nursing homes)	Medicaid, private pay
Acute care (hospitals)	Medicare, private insurance, Medicaid, managed care
Ambulatory care	Medicare, private insurance, Medicaid, private pay
Physicians	
Outpatient clinics	
Community clinics	State and local funds, Medicaid
Adult day care	Medicaid, private pay, county or local government
Home care	Medicare, private insurance, Medicaid, private pay
Medicare-certified	Medicare, private insurance, managed care
Private home care	Private pay, private insurance
Hospice	Medicare, private insurance
Outreach	Internal funding, private pay, Older Americans Act, Medicaid waiver programs
Wellness	Private pay, internal funding
Housing	Private pay, select government programs, HUD for capital for low-income and special populations

Maximize Basic Sources of Funding

The entities participating in the continuum of care should be certain that they are maximizing all potential revenue sources for both the institutions and the individual patients. This means tapping into Medicaid and Veterans Administration eligibility; offering rehabilitation, subacute, and psychiatric services that are still DRG-exempt; and collaborating with public services that may have line-item sources of funding. In keeping with the concept of seamless care, service provider organizations should assist their clients in billing and should coordinate the billing of multiple sources on behalf of the patient.

Recommended Actions

- Enhance the eligibility determination process so that all potential sources of payment are checked for all patients and eligibility applications are completed as quickly as possible.
- Coordinate eligibility determination. If one of the participating entities has verified eligibility, this information should be shared with the other entities to avoid duplication.
- Set up a system wherein a participating entity may check the eligibility status on *all* services when verifying eligibility.
- Implement inpatient services that are DRG-exempt, such as subacute care, rehabilitation, and psychiatry, to use benefits of cost reimbursement to cover staff or services that can be covered by third-party payers.
- If capitation exists, structure risk pools so that the participating providers agree to put part of any excess into services of the continuum that do not have other payment sources.
- Implement a case management program that will help patients and families coordinate services obtained from different funding sources. (See chapter 7.)
- To the extent that there remains any opportunity to do so, maximize cost-shifting to cover services essential to the continuum required by an individual but not covered by other sources.

Explore Secondary Sources of Funding

Providers of basic health services often are less familiar with the variety of service programs and funding sources available through social services, housing, and other funding streams. For example, the Older Americans Act (OAA) funds homemakers, chore services, and friendly visitors, which can be helpful in enabling a frail older person and his or her caregiver to remain at home despite a disability. Another OAA-funded program, Meals-on-Wheels, delivers hot meals to those who are homebound. However, to access such services, the staff of a physician's office must know whom to call to make appropriate arrangements, and few medical offices are set up with such resource staff. Cedars-Sinai Medical Center (CSMC) in Los Angeles applied to the Area Agency on Aging (AAA) to be a certified meal site. It then secured a monthly allocation of meal tickets from the AAA and distributed them through its Senior Resource Center. This provided healthy, low-cost meals to seniors and put excess hospital meal service capacity to use during slow hours, as well as increased CSMC's visibility in the senior community. Unfortunately, few hospitals or nursing homes take advantage of the potential to be an OAA service subcontractor, which brings funding to the institution and, more importantly, needed service to patients and families.

Other types of providers include continuing care retirement communities (CCRCs), which are set up to provide an array of services for residents, often including skilled nursing care, home health, and assisted living, for the entry fee or a discounted fee. To cover the cost of care, the CCRC combines what Medicare will pay for skilled nursing care, what the resident is entitled to as part of her or his buy-in, and what the resident will have to contribute directly.

Recommended Actions

- Investigate federal and state programs that provide health-related services, social services, mental health services, and housing as sources of funding for the continuum.
- Explore local, county, and state programs that fund special services or special populations as sources of funding for the continuum.
- Apply to public sources to become a provider of services found to be needed by continuum clients.

Negotiate with Third-Party Payers

Some of the continuum's services that might not be routinely covered by third-party payers may be covered in special instances if the provider is an effective patient advocate and negotiator. Care for those with AIDS has provided an excellent example of deviations in standard service payment that have evolved into acceptance over the past 10 years. Care at home and in assisted-living facilities that is normally not covered, may be covered for AIDS victims due to special negotiations with the insurer. Service providers must have a legitimate reason for advocating variations in standard coverage to benefit the patient's clinical condition or psychological well-being. In addition, providers must have data demonstrating that the alternative service will be as equally cost-effective as the standard service, or that it will result in an overall cost reduction.

Recommended Actions

- Build databases of costs of the continuum of care, including both individual services and the efficiencies gained through a continuum.
- Establish measures of patient-based outcomes that document the benefit of a seamless continuum of care for the patient.
- Establish measures of utilization and cost outcomes that document the value of the continuum to the participating entities and to the payers.
- Learn which payers are most likely to be flexible and steer patients to them.

Implement Case Management

Many of the services that may be required by people with chronic, long-term illnesses are support services that have funding through an array of public programs. To access these services, a client must apply directly. The role the continuum of care can play is in helping clients apply, advocating on their behalf, monitoring to see if the services are received, and, if received, whether they are adequate. These are functions that can be performed by a case manager. Case managers also can help patients who might have private resources to afford services by persuading the patient, family, or guardian of the services' benefits.

Recommended Actions

- Implement a case management program to help patients access services that are available in the community and for which funding may be available, but which cannot be controlled by the continuum.
- Implement a case management program whereby the case manager has the expertise and authority to deal with third-party payers to negotiate exceptions to standard payment policies to pay for special services.

Initiate Fund-Raising

Some of the continuum services an individual requires may simply not be paid for by third-party sources or may not be accessible due to the individual's categorical limitations (for example, a low-income person who is just above the threshold for Medicaid). Thus, it is helpful to have a backup of private funds available. Henry Mayo Newhall Memorial Hospital (HMNMH), located in the Santa Clarita Valley in southern California, is the only hospital in a valley isolated from Los Angeles by a natural barrier of mountains. Because of all the working couples who had brought their parents there to live, adult day care was an important, but missing, element of the continuum. Financial projections indicated that a day care center would lose money for the hospital. Thus, HMNMH set out to raise an endowment that would provide start-up costs and support ongoing operation. The fund-raising initiative far exceeded expectations, raising more than $400,000 in the then-small community. The endowment provides more than is required to meet the operating shortfall for the day care center and thus has provided funds for other missing services, such as case management. Similarly, the Alzheimer's Association in the greater Tacoma area of Washington State provides scholarships to patients with Alzheimer's disease so that they can afford to attend the local day care and respite programs.

Recommended Actions

- Identify gaps in the continuum or specific activities or programs that could be enhanced by private philanthropy, and apply for one-time or ongoing support.
- Develop a fund-raising initiative specifically to support a designated service, such as an opportunity for a donor to have a program or facility bear his or her name.
- Collaborate with community organizations that represent subsegments of the population needing long-term care (for example, the Alzheimer's Association, American Lung Association, and American Heart Association).
- Educate the foundation board and/or the person responsible for generating contributions to each participating entity about the continuum, its purpose, its benefits to consumers, and the rationale for donating money.

Monitor Demonstrations

Throughout the nation, providers, payers, and policymakers are aware of the negative impact of the fragmentation of financing on health care. A number of demonstration projects are in process that will provide practical knowledge and data on which to base financial calculations and document the benefits of offering flexible services within the context of an organized continuum of care. These projects include the Social Health

Maintenance Organizations (S/HMOs), PACE replications (Programs of All Care for the Elderly), EverCare in Minnesota, Medicaid/Medicare managed care state initiatives, models of chronic care systems funded under a special program of the Robert Wood Johnson Foundation, and state policy projects in California and Minneapolis that are attempting to combine the state funding for several different programs under the control of a single administrative unit with the authority to mingle funds for the benefit of the individual patient.

Recommended Actions

- Monitor (through government reports, professional journals, or presentations) demonstrations at the national, state, and local levels of new ways to organize and finance chronic care.
- Apply to be part of one of these demonstrations.
- Lobby for funding changes at the local, state, and federal levels.

Advocate Private Responsibility

Fragmentation of funding causes fragmentation of service delivery, because services are not available and not affordable. One way to approach afford-ability is to begin now to educate future patients on the need to pay for some of their own health care if they want a comprehensive continuum of care. Many older people continue to believe that Medicare will cover all their health care needs. The American Association of Retired Persons, as well as many local hospitals and aging network organizations, have been trying for years to educate the older population about the limits of Medi-care. Similarly, the companies selling long-term care insurance depend for sales on explaining to potential purchasers the limitations of current third-party health insurance. A major marketing pitch of continuing care retirement communities is that they represent a means for older people to take care of their potential future needs for health care without relying on family or government for financial or functional help. At the federal level, the Kennedy-Kasselbaum legislation authorizes medical IRAs, whereby an individual can build a bank of tax-free funds that could sub-sequently be applied for health care, to cover care costs that are unavail-able through traditional acute care or even long-term care insurance.

Recommended Actions

- Offer seminars on the costs of health care to consumers, includ-ing options for financing their own continuum of care.

- Organize volunteer banks whereby individuals contribute hours of caregiving and social support in exchange for future hours they will receive.
- Continue to lobby state and federal representatives and senators for medical/health IRAs and encourage consumers to use these personal financing vehicles.
- Work with the state hospital, medical, and other professional and trade associations to develop state-sponsored medical IRAs.

Chapter 11

Managed Care

Managed care is one of the primary forces driving efforts to create a seamless continuum of care. However, managed care in and of itself does not mandate a continuum of care, particularly the broad definition used in this book. Managed care's rationale for offering a continuum of care has changed since this structure first emerged on the scene. When closed-panel medical groups and owned hospitals, such as Kaiser Permanente, Group Health Cooperative of Puget Sound, and FHP, were the dominant models of managed care, the emphasis was on providing comprehensive care, including prevention. Today, however, managed care has evolved as a financing arrangement with endless variation in provider structure, including point-of-service plans that resemble fee-for-service arrangements. FHP, which was the first Medicare risk contract health maintenance organization (HMO), threw out its closed-panel, owned-hospital model in 1995, sold its hospitals, and established its physician groups as independent contractors able to contract with any managed care entity. (Subsequently, FHP has been bought by PacifiCare.)

The current rationale for a continuum under managed care arrangements includes the following: The more services a managed care entity provides, the more contracts a provider can have with that entity and thus the more money the provider has the potential to make. Finally, the more services the health plan covers and the more services the provider controls, the greater the potential of each to have flexibility in providing care and meeting the unique needs of individual patients. However, this rationale works only if (1) each of the provider's services is cost-effective on its own and/or the provider is so structured that efficiencies of operation, economies of scale, or substitutability of services are gained by offering multiple services; or (2) a service critical to the continuum from the patient's standpoint is missing from the managed care payment structure but can be covered by the excess revenues from other services that accrue partly because of the existence of that service.

What may be critical to the continuum's success in managed care is not the array of services it provides but, rather, its integrating mechanisms (discussed in chapter 1). For example, in the early 1990s, United Health Plan (a managed care company that operates and manages a managed care health plan) negotiated contracts with a number of community hospitals on the basis that it could save the average 200-bed facility about $1 million per year through better management of just the top ten inpatient diagnoses. Money was made not by offering a continuum of care range of services but, rather, by developing an internal case management program with protocols that served to streamline the provision of patient care.

Once managed care hits an area, it drives up the level of competition. Health plans compete no less than hospitals, physicians, and other health care organizations. In a mature market, providers may have contracts with numerous health plans, each contract having different terms and a different set of contractors and each health plan having its own culture, policies, and operating procedures. Thus, for providers trying to operate their own continuum of care, one managed care contract may complicate matters and several contracts can compound the challenge exponentially.

Managed care is increasingly a financial, regulatory, and marketing health insurance plan, with networks of providers and growing point-of-service plans—models that are not necessarily consistent with the continuum of care framework (particularly as defined in this book). In brief, managed care may indeed be a driving force for creating a continuum of care, but the specific rationale for the continuum must be identified for each individual situation. Furthermore, managed care can help or hinder the existing continuum of care or the one being developed by providers, and in either case, requires more care from the participating entities in the continuum.

Following are the managed care tasks discussed in this chapter:

- Determine the service package.
- Contract for the entire continuum.
- Monitor marketing.
- Integrate the integrating mechanisms.
- Understand the relationships between managed care and the continuum.
- Prepare for changes of contracts.

Determine the Service Package

An example in Los Angeles involving a medical group, a hospital, and an HMO illustrates the need to determine the service package. The medical group touted its broad array of services, including case management, as a continuum of care. The hospital was trying to develop a continuum but did not have exclusive access to the medical group's resources. However, as part of a large corporation that had corporate-offered services, the hospital was able to create its own continuum. Both had a home health agency. The HMO, which held the majority of Medicare enrollees in its service area, contracted with the medical group and the hospital separately. To attract older enrollees, the HMO advertised its one-stop-shopping approach to covering a broad array of services; the hospital and the medical group each marketed its own continuum. Which services were included in the continuum of care? Consumers and providers alike were confused. For example, if a Medicare patient who had been admitted to the hospital subsequently needed home health care, he or she was referred to the hospital's Medicare-certified home health agency, which was included in the contract with the hospital. If the patient returned to visit a physician in the medical group office and needed private home care services, he or she was referred to the medical group's private home health agency because the payment was not constrained by the managed care company. In brief, by contracting with separate providers for the array of services it pays for, the HMO may disrupt continuums of care already put in place by the providers, thus causing fragmentation rather than promoting seamless care.

Recommended Actions

- Decide what services you as a provider have to offer to a health plan and develop contractual rates (including rate options) for each service, but preferably for a package of services.
- Contract explicitly with each health plan for as many services as you have the capacity and financial or service rationale to provide.
- Determine what other providers the health plan contracts with that might affect the services you provide or network with.
- Examine each health plan's marketing materials to understand how they promote your continuum of services; request prior approval of any materials referring explicitly to your services and/or continuum.
- Ask about exclusivity of contracts. (This is a double-edged sword: It works to your advantage when a payer has a large market share but works to your disadvantage when the health plan has only a small portion of the market or a small number of enrollees.)

Contract for the Entire Continuum

Managed care contracting has grown increasingly sophisticated in mature markets as health plans, hospitals, medical groups, and regulators have gained experience. However, in many parts of the country, managed care is still relatively new and mistakes in working with the system are not uncommon. One hospital in a large metropolitan area, for example, purchased a Visiting Nurses Association (VNA) that it had formerly worked with on a affiliated/contract basis. When it came time to renew its contract with the area's major health plan, the hospital did not think about contracting to provide home care as well. When the home health director complained, she was asked what her capitated rate would be. Because the VNA had always contracted with health plans on a per visit basis, she did not have data-based capitation figures available, which caused her political embarrassment. Rather than help calculate the rates, the chief financial officer, who did not understand the home care business and did not want to make the effort to do so, felt vindicated for excluding home health from the contract. As a result, the hospital had to refer its home health clients to another agency for the three-year duration of the contract, and its own home health agency withered.

By now, most hospitals and physicians have established managed care rates. Other providers, however, such as nursing homes or independent home care agencies, may still be in early stages of developing rate structures and contracting terms, particularly in areas where managed care penetration is still low. Thus, some of the entities participating in the continuum may require assistance and leadership from the more experienced participants to develop managed care rates for the entire continuum.

Recommended Actions

- Evaluate every service of the continuum for its potential to contract with a health plan; identify potential weak areas and work collectively to strengthen them.
- Determine the per-service-unit and capitated rate for each service.
- Examine services that can be contracted for through letters of affiliation, contracts, or other network arrangements. A provider having a contract with a health plan may in turn subcontract with other providers in order to maintain control of patient flow.
- Examine the managed care arrangements of your competition. If your organization contracts with a given health plan, are you likely to be referring to your competition for select services of the continuum rather than the continuum in which you choose to participate?

Monitor Marketing

Health plans are experts in marketing. They continuously refine benefit packages, contract with providers, and revise marketing strategies and materials. Providers, on the other hand, tend to put their energies into contracting arrangements and, once negotiations have concluded, to become passive about how the health plan markets their services. A provider organization that already has a continuum of care in place (or is putting one in place) should work with the health plans to maximize the continuum's benefit and to override any marketing that would be detrimental to its continuum.

As an example, one hospital that depended heavily on managed care clients for inpatient occupancy had worked very hard to create a continuum of care. For years, it had been the only hospital contracting with the major HMO targeting its geographic area. However, after several years of success, the hospital began to lose enrollees and discovered that the HMO had contracted with other area hospitals. Rather than marketing this hospital's continuum, the HMO was marketing the competitor's Center of Excellence for Cardiac Care, paying its marketing staff bonuses for small companies and enrollees who signed up for the competing hospital. As a result, the hospital with the continuum was forced to engage in its own major marketing effort, spending its own dollars to promote its continuum and persuade the patients enrolled in the health plan to select it as their hospital of choice.

Recommended Actions

- Learn what each health plan's marketing approach is and determine which plans are most compatible with your organization's philosophy and approach to services.
- Get to know the marketing staff of all the health plans with which you contract.
- Do not depend on the health plan alone to market your services.
- Monitor enrollment and disenrollment from each health plan on an ongoing basis, including enrollment by zip code or other source, and if the health plan offers a choice (and you can acquire the data), monitor the proportion of enrollees that select your organization as their affiliation.
- If your continuum is designed for Medicare, recognize that marketing to seniors is different from marketing to commercial plan enrollees—it tends to be done individually rather than by a group or by employers. To facilitate marketing yourself establish direct relationships with senior organizations and affinity groups.

Integrate the Integrating Mechanisms

As mentioned earlier, managed care's contribution to the continuum of care may be in promoting its integrating mechanisms, rather than a broad array of services. However, this can present its own set of complications. For example, in mature managed care markets, it is common for three separate case management structures to be in place—one each for the HMO, the hospital, and the medical group. Similarly, three or more separate information systems may be operating. Rather than leading to seamless and efficient care, the duplicative systems may in fact increase costs and cause patient and provider confusion.

Recommended Actions

- Find out how each health plan handles case management, information management, quality assurance/utilization review functions, and other operating procedures that will affect your continuum.
- Arrange meetings among provider–entity staff and health plan staff who conduct similar functions, such as marketing, to identify opportunities for collaboration and consistency of message.
- Identify overlapping or duplicate functions that could be eliminated or shared to reduce costs and streamline communication between the health plan and the providers.
- Meet with other providers who contract with the same health plan to search for ways to streamline operations, reduce duplications, and otherwise improve quality or efficiency of care.
- Examine policies that may conflict (for example, one case management program requires personal financial data whereas another specifically prohibits staff from requesting this information). Where irreconcilable differences exist, at least inform staff so that they can communicate consistently and accurately with clients.

Understand the Relationships between Managed Care and the Continuum

It is essential that staff of the continuum organization, including physicians, other clinicians and administrators, and consumers all understand the relationships between the seamless continuum of services offered by the providers and the health plan that will pay for some, but likely not all, of those services. Consumers should be aware that just because services are available from a provider authorized by their health plan, it does not necessarily follow that those services will be paid for by the health plan (or, for that matter, by indemnity insurance). Unfortunately, consumers often fail to read the fine print and sign up for managed care under the assumption that it is a one-policy-covers-all package. As described in chapter 10, the financing of the continuum is currently very fragmented. Thus, in offering a seamless continuum of care, the staff of any entity participating in the continuum must be able to explain to enrollees or patients and families how services can be accessed and paid for.

Recommended Actions

- Develop an educational program for consumers on what a continuum of care is, how it is organized, and how services are paid for.
- Work with health plans in developing marketing materials so that it is clear which services are covered and which are not.
- If your organization has contracts with multiple health plans, simplify contractual terms as much as possible for providers into a chart or quick-reference guide to show which services are paid for, by which health plans, and which provider entities participate for what types of patients. This will help a busy provider quickly determine which services are available for a patient during the patient visit so that the provider can prescribe appropriately, and the patient knows exactly what to expect before leaving the office.

Prepare for Changes of Contracts

If the continuum is based on a number of affiliation agreements or contracts (versus ownership), what happens when one of the organizations you contract with changes health plan affiliations? Can your clients still be referred to that service? Can you find a replacement service?

SCAN, the social health maintenance organization (S/HMO) located in Long Beach, California, had contracted with the same hospital for 10 years when it decided to switch affiliations. The change created a great deal of confusion among its enrollees, who particularly feared they would have to switch physicians. The hospital that had lost the contract still had a vested interest in keeping the seniors enrolled with SCAN because the independent practice association (IPA) that used the hospital retained its contract with SCAN. Thus, because the hospital wanted to support both its physicians and the seniors enrolled in its senior membership program, the program's social worker spent the better part of two months talking with SCAN members and other seniors, conducting information meetings, helping SCAN design new information brochures, and so on. After several years of contracting with the new hospital, SCAN returned to contract with its original hospital.

Recommended Actions

- Make sure that patient loyalty is to your service, as well as to the continuum in which you participate.

- Secure or create and maintain current mailing lists of those health plan enrollees who use your services. If the health plan arrangement changes, you can still contact those enrollees who may prefer to use your services.
- Conduct information sessions for those health plan enrollees eligible to use your services, so that they know to ask for your organization if the health plan arrangement changes but retains some degree of enrollee choice.
- In all affiliation and contract agreements, allow provisions for amicable termination. Better to anticipate the issues of dissolution and deal with them in advance than to face them under crisis.

Chapter 12

Marketing

Marketing is persuading your target audience that you have the product they want at the price they are willing to pay and that you are better than anyone else at meeting their needs. The challenge in marketing a continuum of care is that the term itself means little to the typical consumer. Consumers may recognize and have some understanding of terms such as *comprehensive care* or *full range of services.* Similarly, many professionals still do not relate to the term. Most clinicians are confident about the aspect of care they provide but may not understand all that is required for a full continuum or how their facet of the care process relates to other services needed by patients and their families. Those responsible for marketing may not fully understand what a continuum is and how it differs from the individual services that comprise the medical center or group practice. In brief, marketing a continuum of care requires finding meaningful terminology and educating everyone involved about what the continuum is, what value it has for them, and how it differs from the traditional way care is organized. It also requires finding creative ways to explain the relationships among organizations with different logos, different names, and different ownership.

Recently, one organization that for years had been functioning internally as a coordinated continuum began to struggle with how to present itself to the community so that consumers would understand how they could benefit from the continuum and how they could access its array of services. The organization had 13 different locations in three different counties, with 13 different telephone numbers, multiple prefixes, and two area codes. It found that consumers were deterred from calling because they wanted to avoid a long-distance charge or, in some cases, identified the prefix as remote and assumed the organization did not serve their area. Consumers also were uncertain about which service to call for a specific problem. Thus, the organization determined that a centralized telephone number was essential for it to be perceived as and function as a continuum. The ramifications ranged from hardware issues to public relations issues to staff education. For example, if they wanted to be able to transfer calls from a single location to all 13 sites, an expensive new hardware system would be required. How the telephone was to be answered was another issue: They had to decide on a single name. Who should answer the phone also had to be decided — a receptionist, or a clinician who was professionally capable of triaging clinical calls? All staff had to be informed about the new name, the new single-access system, the job functions of the person answering the telephone, and the telephone call triage process. Moreover, all materials for all services and locations had to be updated with the new telephone number and name.

Following are the marketing tasks discussed in this chapter:

- Educate and involve those responsible for marketing.
- Conduct market research.
- Define the continuum.
- Articulate the relationships of the involved entities.
- Decide on a name and logo.
- Formulate a marketing plan.
- Educate staff.
- Evaluate the continuum.
- Anticipate change.

Educate and Involve Those Responsible for Marketing

The marketing capabilities of the entities participating in the continuum may vary greatly. Multi–health care systems may have large corporate departments that can be accessed, hospitals may have their own departments, a home health agency may have one person whose duties include updating a brochure annually, and a social service agency may have a volunteer fundraising committee but no dedicated marketing staff. In bringing all these entities together, the person responsible for representing each individual participating entity to the community and producing marketing materials should be educated about the continuum. The individual entity will be unable to participate effectively in collective marketing or in the overall positioning of the organization or its separate services unless the marketing staff understands what the continuum is, how it works, and why the entity is participating. Moreover, educating the people responsible for marketing the continuum is a good trial run for educating the rest of the staff about the continuum (and then getting help from the marketers to improve the training).

Recommended Actions

- Identify the person in each participating entity who is responsible for marketing.
- Convene a task force to help develop initial marketing strategies and materials.
- Establish marketing as one of the functions of the continuum management committee, and maintain a subcommittee on marketing if appropriate.
- Educate marketers about each of the participating entities as well as about the total continuum.
- Share marketing materials from each entity with the marketing representatives of the other participating entities so that the marketers learn about each entity's individual services as well as their separate marketing approaches.

Conduct Market Research

Marketing staff are often responsible for collecting market information on a routine basis and also are asked to do special studies. The people responsible for marketing should have the continuum in mind for both types of data. If a single entity is conducting market research, questions pertaining to the continuum should be included. In examining data that have been gathered routinely for years, the marketers may realize that these data are no longer sufficient because they do not answer questions about the continuum. For example, data on market share of inpatient hospitalization, frequently available from state health departments, are increasingly myopic because they tell nothing about what other services of the continuum a patient has used. Similarly, data collected by a hospital on discharge disposition may prove to be too limited to reveal use of the continuum. Although state requirements are likely to be fixed, an individual service entity can often change its own forms to add data fields to collect information oriented toward the continuum perspective. As discussed in chapter 3, the target population of the continuum should be kept in mind in shaping market research sample selection and results analysis.

Recommended Actions

- Develop a set of questions pertinent to the continuum that could be incorporated into individual marketing studies.
- Budget to conduct market research with the defined target population at several points in time.

- Develop a panel of consumers from the target audience who are willing to participate in focus groups or respond to surveys on a regular basis during the continuum's formative years.
- Evaluate routine marketing and market share reports for their applicability to the continuum. If internal, revise them; if external, request revisions or discontinue.
- Develop a method for combining market share information for individual services/payers as a way of getting an overview of market share information for the continuum.
- Work with the marketing and regulatory organizations that compile data to revise their regular reports to pertain to the continuum. For example, hospital utilization data may be compiled by state departments of health services; nursing home utilization data also are reported by the state but by different departments; adult day care utilization may be reported to the state department of social services; moreover, each service may be required to report data in a different unit of analysis. Over time, some of this information can be changed to be more pertinent to integrated systems than to just individual services.

Define the Continuum

The term *continuum* may mean little to consumers or providers. Alternative wording must be used in order to convey something to consumers that they value—for example, "comprehensive services," "one-stop shopping for all your health care needs," or "full range of health care services." In addition, marketing materials must explain how the continuum is different from the standard approach to care and why it offers value to consumers. Just as the term *continuum* may not be meaningful to consumers, its components may be meaningless—or even offensive. For example, many consumers reject the term *case management* on the basis that they (1) want to be thought of as people and not "cases," and (2) do not want to be "managed." Thus, in describing the value of a continuum, professional jargon should be avoided. "We coordinate your care to meet all your needs" is easier for consumers to understand than "We assign case managers to each patient." The mission statement, if there is one, also should be written in terms that can be understood by the lay community. For example, saying that the organization's mission is to "provide and coordinate all the services our families need" is much clearer to consumers than saying that it is to "integrate services through a continuum of care approach."

Recommended Actions

- Conduct focus groups of consumers and professionals to find and/or validate terminology that is simple and meaningful to them.
- Ask recent or current clients what they like about your continuum and draw on their expressions to describe its benefits.

Articulate the Relationships of the Involved Entities

The continuum may be composed of several different organizations brought together in a variety of arrangements. Describing this to consumers may be complex, particularly if each participating entity engages heavily in marketing campaigns of its own. The organizations comprising the continuum may choose to promote themselves as "partners in serving the community," "joining together to meet all your needs," "a network that coordinates care," "service providers working together to offer high-quality, comprehensive care," or other similar phrases. Whatever language is chosen should be as clear as possible about how the service providers are linked in the continuum, what the relationship is (if any) to payers, and how the continuum approach benefits the client. The task of articulating the relationship among the participating entities is particularly challenging for continuums that are organized through affiliation and for networks; ownership models may be somewhat easier to explain to external consumers.

Recommended Actions

- Decide with your partners how to describe the relationship in a way that each participant finds acceptable, then market-test the terminology.
- Educate staff about the relationship among the participating entities and inform them of the language and marketing materials being used with consumers.

Decide on a Name and Logo

The continuum may develop its own name and logo. If the continuum's primary purpose is to increase market share through enrollment of individuals or through contracting, this would help with market recognition and may be a central part of a marketing strategy. Alternatively, if its primary purpose is to increase efficiency of patient transfers and to enhance quality, marketing the continuum with a single name and logo may not be necessary.

Arriving at a single name and logo may be difficult if many entities from different organizations are involved, each with a distinct name and logo. Even within the same organization, different departments or units often have totally separate marketing materials, individual logos, and distinct colors. Trying to coordinate marketing within an organization, let alone among several organizations, is a challenge. Moreover, existing names may have great consumer loyalty, whereas a new name would have no name recognition. When Fairview and The Ebenezer Society, in Minneapolis, merged, they agreed to carry both names on many of their services, at least for the short run, because each had a strong market recognition that no new name could duplicate.

Recommended Actions

- Evaluate the benefit of a new name and logo.
- Select a name that conveys the meaning of the continuum in terms understandable to the lay community.
- Find a compromise between the name recognition needs of the continuum and those of its participating entities. For example, adopt a common logo and color scheme to indicate participation in the continuum but continue to use the individual names of the participating entities.
- Gather marketing materials from other continuums in the market and in other markets.
- Market-test name, logo, colors, and materials with consumers and with staff of each of the participating entities.

Formulate a Marketing Plan

Once the basics of name, logo, definition, relationships and access numbers, and other operating procedures have been determined, the other components of the continuum's marketing plan must be developed. This should include a wide array of activities in addition to standard promotional materials. The marketing plan should reflect the continuum's goals and objectives, and should include a budget. In the event that the individual entities are unwilling to give up their separate marketing efforts, the collaborative marketing plan must be designed so as to complement, rather than compete with, the separate marketing plans. Finally, although in some instances marketing may be important to recruit participants to implement the continuum, in most instances the entities comprising the continuum already exist and have clients. Thus, it is preferable to first get the continuum under way as a seamless, integrated system per se, and then engage in marketing. This allows time to ensure that the system can deliver what it promises, rather than making grand promises only to discover that operational details have not been worked out.

Recommended Actions

- Formulate a plan for marketing the continuum, developed by or with input from the people in each participating entity responsible for marketing.
- Review the marketing plans of the individual entities to look for opportunities, such as calendar event dates, and conflicts, such as different terminology.
- Develop a budget for marketing. This may be an aspect that the individual entities overlooked when they agreed to collaborate. Moreover, if collaboration is primarily through affiliation rather than ownership or creation of a new corporation, a formula will need to be established to assess each entity for its contribution to the collective marketing plan.
- Include in the plan marketing to other providers and community organizations, as well as consumers.

Educate Staff

A key component of marketing the continuum is educating the staff of the individual entities about what the continuum is, how it works, and why it adds value to the organization and their own activities. Internal staff can make or break the continuum's efficient operation and consumer perceptions of it; thus, internal marketing within and among the staffs of the participating entities may be just as important as marketing to the community. One organization addressed the issue of physician awareness by creating a prescription pad listing the many services offered through the continuum. All the physician had to do was check a box, which keyed nurses to call for referrals to the services identified. Although the people responsible for marketing may think of their activities as primarily client- and externally oriented, their expertise can be applied internally as well. Particularly in small organizations that may not have separate staff dedicated to employee education or marketing, combining the efforts of those responsible for these functions through the continuum entities can bring together an important resource for marketing.

For example, one medical group at risk for primary care, secondary care, and home care assigns case managers to guide its complicated patients through the system, and one trigger of the system is hospitalization. When a particular patient was hospitalized, she met the nurse case manager who was responsible for streamlining her inpatient care. The nurse was experienced with clinical pathway management, but new to the hospital and unfamiliar with the medical group's internal operations. The patient was confused about how the medical group case manager and the hospital case manager differed, and the hospital case manager did not know what the medical group case managers did, let alone how to explain the differences in their roles to the patient or her family. This left the patient wondering who was indeed responsible for coordinating her care. The need for internal marketing of the continuum was clear.

Recommended Actions

- At the outset of the continuum, or when major steps in evolution occur, conduct special joint educational programs for everyone from all participating entities.
- Conduct educational orientations in conjunction with regularly scheduled staff meetings.
- Bring together people holding similar positions in the various participating entities to learn how the continuum will affect their jobs and their working relationships with each other. For example, admission clerks would come together to problem-solve issues such as streamlining the admission process. They also would learn how to explain to patients how the continuum works, so that if patients were admitted to one of the participating entities, they would not have to answer all information for all the other entities in the continuum (yet the information would be available to all the continuum's providers).
- Incorporate information on the continuum into new employee orientation and in-service education to accommodate staff turnover.

Evaluate the Continuum

The state of the art of constructing and operating seamless continuums of care is sufficiently new that consensus has not yet been reached on valid evaluation criteria. The government agencies and private quality monitors still focus on individual services rather than the continuum. Nonetheless, many organizations do patient follow-up surveys as part of their ongoing market research. This presents an opportunity to evaluate the continuum at very low, if any, marginal cost to the participating entities. Regardless of external criteria, at minimum, the organizations participating in the continuum can ask similar questions of their staff and patients, and compare results. In addition, as mentioned previously, a separate marketing budget should be allocated that includes funds for conducting surveys or focus groups specifically on continuum issues. Collectively or individually, participating entities can evaluate the extent to which the definition of the continuum is understood and find out subjectively, as well as objectively, if the continuum's organizational arrangements have made a difference in the care that staff provide or patients and families receive.

Recommended Actions

- Compile the types of staff and patient evaluations done by each of the entities involved in the continuum. Look for overlaps and opportunities to add comparable questions across entities.
- Conduct a market test to assess recognition of the continuum's name, logo, and value.
- Set up a short-term task force to develop criteria and ongoing methods to evaluate the continuum from the patient, family, clinician, and support staff perspectives.

Anticipate Change

At the present time in the evolution of the health care delivery system, relationships seem to change daily in dramatic ways. Alliances come and go; mergers are proposed; proposed mergers fall apart; provider affiliations change as new health plans enter the market; and so on. Thus, the marketing of the continuum of care must be prepared for change. Thousands of unused brochures may need to be pitched, and the dollars spent on them lost. Organizers may schedule health fairs involving all the participating entities a year in advance, only to find out 3 weeks before the event that several of the key players have merged or are affiliated with the competition. Similarly, new entities may have joined the continuum, and loose affiliations may have been tightened by contracts or purchase. There is no way to enter into a collaborative relationship with zero risk. However, there are ways to minimize risk and to maximize the ability to constructively manage the unexpected dissolution of the relationship.

Recommended Actions

- Include cancellation clauses in all formal agreements. This is the responsibility of top management, not marketing. However, the existence of such clauses should prompt each participating entity to be prepared to think through what would cause a cancellation and how it would be handled by the organization operationally. This makes the related public relations/marketing efforts much easier.

- Develop marketing materials and strategies that allow for positive as well as negative changes in the continuum. For example, use a master folder with inserts for each participating entity, but do not stagger the inserts; in the event that one entity drops out or two merge, that would create a noticeable gap.
- Focus on making the operations work smoothly before doing any marketing to avoid touting benefits that may be changed once the continuum is implemented. Getting operations under way prior to marketing provides the opportunity to identify problems that should be resolved and those that may be unresolvable, without negatively affecting marketing.

Chapter 13

Evaluation

Once a continuum of care is created, or is in process, it is time to evaluate its impact. Do patients have access to a full range of services? Can they obtain services when they need them? Are efficient and easy transfers among services being achieved? Are patients being referred within the system? What are the reasons for referrals outside the system? Are the costs of the continuum less or more than those of individual services? Do staff think of themselves as a single system? Does the continuum have market recognition? Can one entity negotiate managed care at-risk contracts that include all elements of the continuum? Has patient, family, provider, and payer satisfaction increased or decreased? Does the continuum organization improve quality of care? Are the mission, goals, and objectives, as specified during the initial planning of the continuum, being met?

The techniques and criteria for evaluating the delivery of health care are evolving and changing. This is ever more true for the continuum. Each of its many individual services must be evaluated. Moreover, the continuum integrating mechanisms must be evaluated, both individually and for their collective effect. All four of the basic integrating mechanisms used in the definition of the continuum in chapter 1—inter-entity management, care coordination, integrated information systems, and integrated financing—are still being developed and tested. Complete consensus on form is lacking, let alone on outcomes and measurement criteria. Finally, the operations and outcome of the overall continuum must be assessed to determine if the whole is greater than the sum of the parts.

To date, no external, objective, validated data bank exists for measuring and comparing achievement of a seamless continuum of care across organizations or over time. Evaluating the continuum implies knowing what it is, having explicit goals and objectives, and having baseline data. What does *seamless* mean in operating terms? Chapter 1 offers a definition of a continuum of care, but how each continuum defines itself will differ. And, as noted in the introduction to this book, many organizations use the terminology of a seamless continuum of care without great attention to what it means from the standpoint of the patient, provider, or payer. Thus, evaluation must begin with the entities participating in the continuum referring to their original goals and objectives.

Evaluation of the continuum is hindered by the same fragmentation that characterizes the rest of the U.S. health care delivery system. For some services, such as hospitals, sophisticated and well-established mechanisms for evaluation are in place (although they, too, continue to evolve). For example, the Joint Commission on Accreditation of Healthcare Organizations (JCAHO) is a well-developed and nationally recognized body that accredits 80 percent of the hospitals in the United States. (See table 13-1 for a sample list of services and the bodies that accredit them.) Most states also have well-defined licensing requirements for hospitals. In its role as a major payer of services, the federal government has explicit conditions of participation that hospitals must meet in order to participate in Medicare and Medicaid. In contrast, for other services, evaluation criteria are scarce. For example, assisted living facilities, which are still being defined, are not even licensed in some states, let alone regulated. Accreditation is done by the American Association of Homes and Services for the Aging, but to date, relatively small numbers of facilities have undertaken the process. Adult day care programs are neither licensed nor regulated in all states. Because adult day care is not reimbursed by Medicare

Table 13-1. Examples of Nongovernmental Agencies Accrediting Health Care Organizations

Service/Program	Accreditation Agency
Hospitals	JCAHO
Ambulatory care (including clinics and medical groups)	Association for Accreditation of Ambulatory Care and Community Health and Accreditation Program
Nursing homes	JCAHO
Home health	National HomeCaring Counsel JCAHO
Hospice	JCAHO
Retirement communities	Continuing Care Accreditation Commission American Association of Homes and Services for the Aging
Medical groups w/capitation	The Medical Quality Commission
Health plans and networks	National Commission for Quality Assurance

and by only select states under Medicaid, the Older Americans Act, or social service agencies, there are no uniform federal regulations. Standards for adult day care were developed by the National Council on Aging in the late 1980s, but there is no accrediting body. Thus, implementation of the procedures and criteria for evaluating the continuum falls on a varied base. Although some continuums are primarily within a single parent organization, others are network models, which makes uniform evaluation all the more difficult.

Nonetheless, evaluation initiatives have begun. The JCAHO began to offer accreditation for networks in 1994. Gillies and colleagues conducted a longitudinal study of major health care systems, from which they identified characteristics of integrated systems they considered to be successful.[1] Coddington and colleagues have done case studies of large medical groups and examined factors of successful hospital–medical group integration.[2]

The National Chronic Care Consortium (NCCC) has developed an instrument for planning and measuring systems readiness for integration called Self-Assessment for Systems Integration (SASI).[3] SASI comprises nine components that "assist health care providers and systems to conceptualize, plan, implement, and measure the degree to which they are providing integrated chronic care." These areas include: governance, management structures and strategies, information systems, financing, services array, high-risk populations, disability prevention, seamless care, and client involvement. Each module of the instrument contains specific criteria by which to evaluate that aspect of the organization's move toward integration. SASI has been beta-tested, and it became available for purchase in 1996. The next step planned by the NCCC will be to gather and compare data on systems across sites and to refine the instrument on the basis of the feedback from users.

To date, few baseline data or trend data are available on organizational integration. How individual service evaluation criteria relate to system evaluation criteria remains to be explicated. Overall, conceptual agreement on evaluation criteria for the continuum and validity in measurement techniques and data collection procedures remain in the early stages of development.

Following are the quality and evaluation tasks discussed in this chapter:

- Evaluate individual continuum services.
- Look at separate evaluations already in place.
- Measure continuum uniqueness.
- Measure continuum objectives.
- Allocate resources for collective evaluation.
- Maximize value for marketing.
- Design for the long term.

Evaluate Individual Continuum Services

As noted previously, the services comprising the continuum may be evaluated individually through professional accreditation, licensure, or certification. However, undergoing these reviews is both costly and time-consuming. Before the continuum commits itself to yet more evaluation, it would be helpful to find out by whom and by what criteria elements of the continuum are already being evaluated. Whether entities are participating in more than one continuum also should be noted.

Recommended Actions

- Find out which of the continuum's services are licensed, certified, or accredited. Delineate the external authority, the costs, the time frame, the evaluation process, and the criteria.
- Ask the entities participating in the continuum to share their licensing/accreditation/certification results. (This will be a real indicator of trust.)
- Look for disparities in accreditation of the participating entities. (For example, nursing homes do not seek JCAHO accreditation because of the cost.) Assess the value of having the participants in the continuum pool budgets to get all components accredited/licensed/certified.

Look at Separate Evaluations Already in Place

Apart from what is required by regulatory or accrediting authorities, the entities participating in the continuum may have their own evaluations in place, such as regular or occasional patient satisfaction surveys. Each entity may want to maintain its own evaluation for its own purposes but also be willing to add questions pertinent to the continuum of care. Alternatively, participating entities may be willing to pool their resources to design an evaluation that measures continuum issues and adds secondary questions to benefit the individual components. In the case of one continuum, its hospital, medical group, home health agency, and health plan found that they were all conducting regular patient satisfaction surveys of basically the same pool of patients. By joining together, they reduced expenses, increased response rate, and were able to include questions that reflected the entire patient experience rather than just one aspect of it.

Recommended Actions

- Ascertain what evaluations are done internally by each of the participating entities and the purposes for which they are done.

- Collect and compare evaluation instruments, data reports, target population, methodology, frequency, and dissemination of evaluations done by individual participating entities.
- Look for opportunities and methods to conduct joint evaluations, and document the benefits of collaboration (such as decreased costs, increased response rate, and improved patient satisfaction).

Measure Continuum Uniqueness

Each continuum is unique, with its own goals and objectives, participating entities, clients, and other features. Thus, regardless of what external evaluation criteria and processes may be available, each continuum needs to consider how it will measure its success in ways that are explicable to its relevant stakeholders.

Recommended Actions

- Have the executive team that first planned collaboration and articulated the continuum's vision, goals, and objectives also specify the evaluation processes and criteria and assume ongoing responsibility for monitoring the evaluation process and findings.
- Convene a separate task force to develop common and shared evaluation methods and criteria.
- During the continuum's planning phase, articulate the evaluation criteria and methods at the outset as one technique for explaining goals and objectives to staff, governance, and clients. Gaining consensus on evaluation among the participating entities will help solidify trust (or reveal the lack thereof).
- Establish an evaluation process that has a prespecified means of using the findings to improve the continuum. What if results do not meet objectives? Does the continuum fall apart, or does it have the commitment and process to improve?

Measure Continuum Objectives

Each participating entity should consider the operational implications for measuring continuum objectives. As is often the case, what sounds good in principle may be difficult to implement, particularly if it requires gathering data from others who have not been involved in the process. For example, in one continuum, the chief executive officers of the participating services agreed to track and measure the source of all referrals to their organizations and the direction of all discharge referrals to other organizations on a monthly basis, and then calculate the percentage of patients both maintained in and lost to the continuum. They discovered that each service provider maintained a different referral source and discharge format. For example, some coded generic organizations (such as home health) and some recorded specific organizations (such as VNA); not all used identical names for the same agency (for example, Visiting Nurses, Visiting Nurses Association, VNA); some tallied monthly, others weekly; the department or person recording referral source was usually not the person recording discharge disposition; different forms for admission/discharge were required by different regulators, making extra work to code information in a new format. The organizations had to conduct a special study during the planning phase of their continuum to gather agreed-on baseline data. Implementing a system that would gather the desired data routinely required extensive education of all staff involved, a task force to develop consensus on data elements and format, several months to implement and validate the data collection and reporting system, and an ongoing commitment to the extra effort required to collect the information that would enable them collectively to measure the use of their continuum. Thus, measurement requires both consensus in concept and cooperation in actual implementation.

Recommended Actions

- In delineating the measures to be used to evaluate the continuum, each participating entity should be specific about what data it will use, the source of the data, the data elements, and the format. This should be shared with the board and executive management of each participating entity for their acceptance.
- Convene a short-term task force to review the data each participant gathers and then evaluate how comparable they are and what must be done to compile them into a report that addresses the whole continuum and the operating issues of seamlessness.
- At the outset of continuum development, ask the senior executives representing each of the participating entities, including the physicians, to determine what, if any, routine reports they agree to collect and share with each other concerning the continuum's overall operation. They could then delegate to the short-term task force the responsibility for determining how to gather the information and for working out the mechanics for doing so.
- As part of ongoing operations, incorporate mechanisms to respond to evaluation findings. The continuum of care director or the inter-entity management team may have the responsibility and authority to act on some types of evaluation findings; the executive management team may be responsible for others.

Allocate Resources for Collective Evaluation

To conduct any type of evaluation requires resources. As noted previously, much effort and extensive resources may already be required of each participating entity for the individual accreditation/certification/licenses required. To participate in the overall evaluation, each organization may be asked to commit even more. For example, an entity participating in several continuums, either different networks or continuums for different target populations, may find itself asked to participate in several evaluation initiatives, placing an even greater demand on its resources. Yet, if the total continuum is not evaluated, over time, the participating entities or even individual professionals may wonder if it is worth the extra effort required for collaboration.

Recommended Actions

- As part of continuum planning, gain commitment from the participating entities to share in the overall evaluation.
- Identify ways that direct costs or staff time can be saved by consolidating evaluation activities.
- Focus evaluation on the most important elements and those of greatest interest to all participating entities; do not try to evaluate everything all the time.
- Stage evaluations. For example, survey patients one year and providers another. Establish a minimum annual fund for evaluation and use it over time to assess different aspects of the continuum.
- Seek out universities to partner with on the research. Faculty and students looking for projects often offer their free or low-cost services in exchange for real-world experience or the opportunity to publish a paper.

Maximize Value for Marketing

Evaluation results can be a powerful marketing tool. As noted several times, consumers are unlikely to understand the meaning or implications of a continuum of care, let alone descriptions of esoteric research. Therefore, any type of evaluation results must be couched in terms the lay public can understand.

Recommended Actions

- Bring together evaluation researchers and marketers (for example, on a task force, on a standing committee, or through biannual

lunches) to ensure that they are gathering information of interest
to consumers and that marketing is using the evaluation findings
to enhance consumer loyalty and to recommend operational en-
hancements to the participating entities and to the continuum of
care management team.
- Encourage those designing the evaluation to coordinate with
  research being done by the marketing departments of the participating entities. They may find that questions pertinent to the
  continuum can be incorporated at no or low cost into surveys or
  focus groups already being organized and paid for by other components of provider or payer entities.

Design for the Long Term

Over time, trends can reveal progress and problems with the operations
of the continuum. As noted previously, no central source has begun to
track and record performance data on the seamless continuum of care.
Thus, it is up to each organization to do so on its own. Moreover, new
evaluation methodologies may need to be developed to measure the continuum, such as the case of SASI. New instruments, new scales, and
new criteria may appear and need to be incorporated into the continuum's evaluation. As the continuum expands and changes over time,
additional modifications may be made to the evaluation to accommodate those changes.

As an example, a rural area that had previously not had an adult
day care program available referred all clients who had any potential of
benefiting from socialization to the lunch meal program at the local senior
center. However, when the adult day care program opened, referrals to
the senior center suddenly dropped. The evaluation methodology had
to be expanded to include the adult day care program, and reports had
to be modified to explain the drop in referrals to the senior center.

Recommended Actions

- Include participation in the ongoing evaluation as one of the
  requirements for new entities joining the continuum, including
  specifying data coding and data collection procedures.
- Gain commitment from the executive management team responsible for the evaluation to ensure that resources and mechanisms
  are in place to have ongoing monitoring and adoption of new
  advances in health care evaluation technology.
- Submit data that are not deemed private in articles to professional
  journals or present them at professional society conferences in

order to solicit feedback from others working in the integration arena.

- Periodically bring in outside experts to review the evaluation design and findings. This will help prevent the evaluation from being co-opted by the continuum.

References

1. Gillies, R., Shortell, S., Anderson, D., Mitchell, J., and Morgan, K. Conceptualizing and measuring integration: findings from the Health Systems Integration Study. *Hospital and Health Services Administration* 38:4, Winter 1993.

2. Coddington, D., Moore, K., and Fischer, E. *Integrated Health Care: Reorganizing the Physician, Hospital and Health Plan Relationship.* Englewood, CO: Center for Research in Ambulatory Health Care Administration, 1994.

3. National Chronic Care Consortium. *Self-Assessment for Systems Integration Tool.* Bloomfield, MN: NCCC, 1996.

Part Three

Case Studies

Chapter 14

The Carle Clinic Association

Cheryl Schraeder, RN, PhD, and Paul Shelton, EdD

Carle Clinic, a large multispecialty clinic located in Urbana, Illinois, is a cornerstone for geriatric services in east central Illinois and western Indiana. It was founded in 1931 by two physicians, Thomas Rogers and Hugh Davison, who wanted to transplant the concept of multispecialty group practice they had experienced at the Mayo Clinic to central Illinois. More than 60 years later, Carle Clinic patients have access to primary care and virtually all types of specialty care and advanced procedures, conveniently located close to home. The clinic provides area residents with the resources of a comprehensive medical center and a full complement of related services.

The Carle Clinic Association is one of the largest private physician group practices in the country, serving nearly 2,000 patients daily. It is a large multispecialty practice with more than 280 physicians practicing in 50 medical and surgical specialties and subspecialties. The Carle Organizations include the Carle Clinic, the Carle Foundation, and the Carle Foundation Hospital, a 300-bed non-for-profit hospital. Together, they have provided sophisticated health care services to more than 8 million patients residing in predominantly rural areas. (See figure 14-1 for a map of the clinic's primary catchment area.)

Rationale for Serving Seniors

Most of Carle Clinic's special programs for seniors have been developed during the 1990s. This new thrust was motivated by the reality of an increasing older population and decreasing payment from Medicare.

Clinic administrators have focused their efforts on discovering new strategies to compensate for shrinking Medicare dollars and to adjust

Cheryl Schraeder is head of and Paul Shelton is a research analyst at Carle Clinic Association's Health Systems Research Center in Urbana, Illinois.

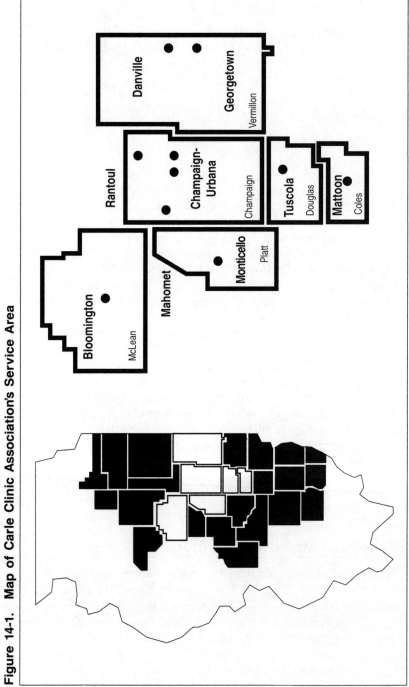

Figure 14-1. Map of Carle Clinic Association's Service Area

to evolving requirements of other payers. Anticipating that managed care is the payment mechanism of the future, the clinic has been experimenting with new ways to deliver health care services to its geriatric patients.

Carle Clinic has several goals in providing care to seniors, including:

- To be cost-effective in managing the care for all patients/clients, especially seniors
- To deliver coordinated services for seniors, including referrals to community agencies
- To maintain seniors in the most appropriate setting

Carle Clinic Services

The breadth and depth of services offered and owned by Carle Clinic is impressive. Along with the acute care hospital and 13 branch clinics, the clinic offers a geriatric evaluation clinic, a geriatric hospital consult service, a geriatric outpatient clinic, nursing home rounding service, the Carle Hospice (Medicare-certified), the Carle HomeCare (Medicare-certified), Carle Medical Supply, The Carle Arbours (195-bed nursing home), Windsor of Savoy (retirement community), pharmacological drug trials, nurse case management programs, and Health Alliance Medical Plans (an HMO that includes supplemental insurance for Medicare patients).

Carle Clinic Mission and Marketing Approach

Carle's mission is to provide superior health care and related services to its patients. To accomplish this, the Carle philosophy highlights the benefits of keeping its seniors healthy and living at home through health management programs, rather than offering only sick care. The clinic regularly monitors patient satisfaction through surveys, and it incorporates community and provider focus groups as part of its marketing and public relations efforts.

The Clinic's Operations

The following subsections describe Carle's principal operations.

Patient Flow

With Urbana as the referral center and major hub for inpatient and specialized care, the Carle system is designed to provide primary care to patients throughout central Illinois and western Indiana through a network of 13 branch clinics. (See figure 14-1.) Each branch clinic is staffed with primary care clinicians and uses local community services and networks with local providers to create smaller "hubs" of service that serve areas within a 30-mile radius of the branch. Referrals for specialty care come to Carle from a network of 2,000 physicians, with more than 50 percent of Carle patients coming from outside Urbana.

Staffing

Two-thirds of Carle physicians specialize in primary care. Fifty medical and surgical specialties and subspecialties also are represented. Several of the 55 primary care physicians (both internists and family practitioners) have received board certification in geriatrics through the subspecialty exam. More than three-quarters of the physicians have their offices in the main clinic in Urbana.

Carle Clinic is staffed by 210 registered nurses, 43 nurse practitioners, and 15 nurse case managers. These mid-level practitioners are critical to certain components of the clinic's gerontology programs.

The Clinic's Geriatric Programs

The nursing home rounding service benefits patients in nursing homes, nursing home staff, physicians, and families. Three geriatric nurse practitioners follow patients placed in nursing homes, whether for short-term recovery or ongoing care. Although the physician continues to visit the patient, the nurses do so more frequently and become a vital communication link among physician, family, and nursing home staff. They also instruct nursing home staff in appropriate care, thus enhancing the overall quality of care available to all patients of the nursing home. The three nurses who are part of the rounding service go to nursing homes throughout the community, wherever Carle Clinic patients are referred.

The geriatric evaluation clinic provides comprehensive medical evaluation of seniors by a physician. The goal of the evaluation is to help seniors maintain or improve their functional status so that they can remain in, or return to, their preferred living arrangements.

The geriatric hospital consult service assists seniors who are about to be discharged from the hospital to a nursing home. Geriatric nurse practitioners and physicians consult on the follow-up treatment and care that seniors will need in this new environment.

Case Management

As the number of older patients requiring supportive services has increased, Carle Clinic has developed models of nursing-based, case-managed health care to support individuals living in the community. These case management models provide in-home nursing coordination and referral to community-based services. Case management services include the initial screening of potential clients, in-home assessment, care planning and delivery, the arrangement and coordination of services, health and service utilization monitoring, and the consistent evaluation of needs and services.

One full-time nurse manages approximately 100 patients, helping to coordinate their overall health care needs, including community services. Many seniors do not use available community services, even though they are paid for and available, because they are unaware of them. The nurse case manager handles high-risk seniors who need preventive attention and individual reassurance more than medical care.

The Community Nursing Organization (CNO), funded by the Health Care Financing Administration (HCFA), is a nurse-managed primary care provider organization for Medicare recipients designed to provide home health care and selected outpatient ambulatory care services through a capitated payment system. Nurse case managers provide in-depth assessments, individualized care plans, authorization for needed health services, referrals to appropriate community-based services, and continual monitoring of care.

Partners in Care, originally a demonstration project sponsored by the John A. Hartford Foundation, links primary care physicians, their office staff, and nurse case managers in running a clinic-based program that targets "at-risk" seniors and their caregivers. Using a team approach, nurse case managers provide in-home assessment, care planning, monitoring, and evaluation, in addition to reviewing plans with physicians to optimize care and better integrate Carle's health care delivery system. By 1996, the program had served approximately 730 clients.

Information Systems

The Carle Clinic/Carle Foundation tracks patients through integrated patient records. Each patient has a single identification number, so records are consistent and accessible throughout the system whether the patient comes into the hospital, the main clinic, or a branch clinic.

The case management programs are built around an integrated patient record, using computerized relational databases designed to track the various stages of client information—from the earliest subject selection stage through the intake process, interviews, assessments, care plans, problem lists, and health care service utilization, to eventual attrition from the program. The benefits of such a system include instant, on-line access to any part of the client record; automatic generation of project status reports that collate information; automated determination of upcoming patient contact; and ease of access for data analyses. Any of the data stored in the databases can be readily analyzed by statistical and financial packages.

Financing/Reimbursement/Budgeting

Revenue for the Carle Clinic is approximately 40 percent managed care, with the remainder being a mix of private insurance, public funds, and private pay. The clinic takes a realistic approach when starting any new initiative. It depends on grant moneys and outside funding to develop or experiment with new ways of delivering care. If the program is beneficial and can be made cost-effective, and if a payment source is found or established, the clinic will evaluate the service for integration into its regular health care delivery system.

Administrative Structure

The Carle organizations consist of the Carle Clinic Association and the Carle Foundation. The latter is a not-for-profit holding company that owns and operates Carle Foundation Hospital and a number of vertically integrated health care businesses. Its sister corporation, Carle Clinic Association, is a for-profit, 280-physician multispecialty group practice that wholly owns Health Alliance Medical Plans, Inc., a domestic stock insurance company that operates a 100,000 plus–member HMO, as well as offering PPO and other insurance products. (See figure 14-2.)

The policy-making body of the clinic is a board of governors composed of six physicians elected for staggered three-year terms. The senior administrative team includes a physician chief executive officer (CEO), a physician assistant to the CEO, a physician medical director, and two nonphysician administrators responsible for ongoing operations and management.

The clinic physicians are organized under a framework of nine major departments (medicine, surgery, anesthesia, pediatrics, radiology, pathology/laboratory, family practice, obstetrics and gynecology, and emergency medicine) within which there are a number of divisions with physician heads. The head of each department serves on the department head council, which provides recommendations to the board of governors on policy and physician governance issues.

Relationships with Other Agencies

The Carle organizations deal with a vast network of health care providers. They contract with more than 20 hospitals, 350 physicians, 150 pharmacies, and 60 community health care and social agencies to bring services to a geographically dispersed senior population.

Figure 14-2. Carle Clinic Association's Organizational Structure

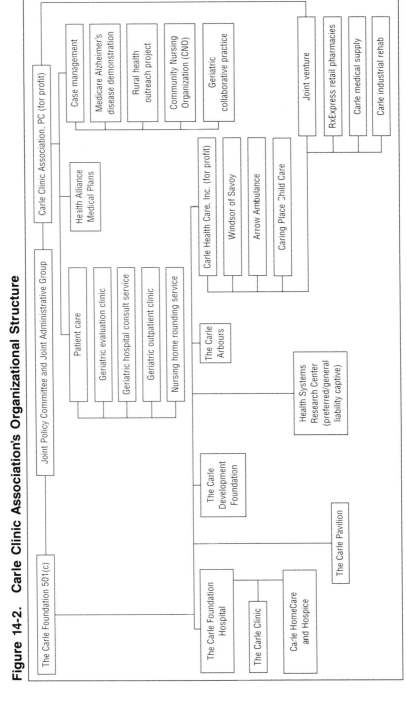

Source: Mchamet Clinic, Mohamet, IL. Reprinted with permission.

Evaluation

Geriatric programs meet family, patient, provider, and societal needs if the services:

- Coordinate the care of seniors
- Meet assessed patient/caregiver needs and problems
- Mobilize appropriate resources to meet patient/caregiver needs
- Support the formal and informal caregiving network
- Are continually evaluated and improved based on expected patient, caregiver, and program goals and outcomes

Patient Example

Mrs. Walters is a 73-year-old senior living alone on the family farm in western Champaign County. Although generally healthy, she suffers from mild hypertension. Returning from the barn one winter morning, she slips on the icy front steps to her house and breaks her hip. Her daughter finds her and calls her physician at the Carle branch clinic in Mohamet, Illinois. The doctor tells the daughter to take her mother by ambulance to Carle Foundation Hospital, where he will meet them.

Once admitted, Mrs. Walters is operated on by one of the clinic's orthopedic surgeons, and a case manager is assigned to her case. The geriatric hospital consult service assists Mrs. Walters as she is discharged for rehabilitation from the hospital to The Carle Arbours, a 195-bed nursing home. A geriatric nurse practitioner follows her as part of the nursing home rounding service.

The nurse case manager works with Mrs. Walters, her primary care physician, her orthopedic surgeon, the geriatric nurse practitioner, and the discharge planner at the Arbours to develop a plan for her return home. Once there, Carle HomeCare provides in-home care for Mrs. Walters. The case manager arranges for a homemaker from a local agency to come in two hours a day, three days a week to help Mrs. Walters. Mrs. Walters gets around with the help of first a walker and then a cane, both supplied by Carle Medical Supply. She also is equipped with a Carle Home Alert communication system that will enable her to call for help in the event of future problems.

As Mrs. Walters improves, her nurse case manager continues to provide in-home assessment, care planning, monitoring, and evaluation, working as a team with her primary care physicians and their staff to optimize care at an appropriate level.

Chapter 15

Mercy Medical

Charles Kondis

Mercy Medical is a multiservice health care provider located in Daphne, Alabama. It was founded in 1949 by the Sisters of Mercy as a long-term care facility. A 137-bed inpatient facility still stands on the original site. As an organization, Mercy Medical has grown and evolved into a unique continuum of care with services ranging from acute medical rehabilitation to residential living options. Starting as a small inpatient facility, it has expanded to eight sites throughout Baldwin and Mobile Counties in southwestern Alabama, including the city of Mobile. (See figure 15-1.)

Mission

Mercy Medical's continuum of care is rooted in its mission. Simply stated, Mercy Medical offers a continuum of care through an emphasis on programs designed to encourage independence. The vision statement for the current strategic plan echoes this commitment to the delivery of a number of specialized services and programs in various locations throughout Mobile and Baldwin Counties.

Development of the continuum has always been needs-based, meeting first the health care and now the residential needs of the community, particularly its older citizens. The driving force of Mercy Medical is its belief that the frail elderly and others who are medically compromised can have some level of independence; can achieve a level of wellness under adverse circumstances; and can remain in control of their lives and their decision making ability. Through experience, Mercy Medical has found that older adults prefer small organizations and settings, and prefer to remain close to their local neighborhoods.

Charles Kondis is director of governance and strategic planning at Mercy Medical in Daphne, Alabama.

The various programs within Mercy Medical's continuum have developed and evolved at various times in its history, but it has been the commitment of its board and administration to pursue an intensive rehabilitation model, rather than a traditional nursing home model, that has made the difference. Although, over time, the continuum has been expanded to include new programs and services, it has always remained rooted in the medical model.

Figure 15-1. Map of Mercy Medical's Service Locations

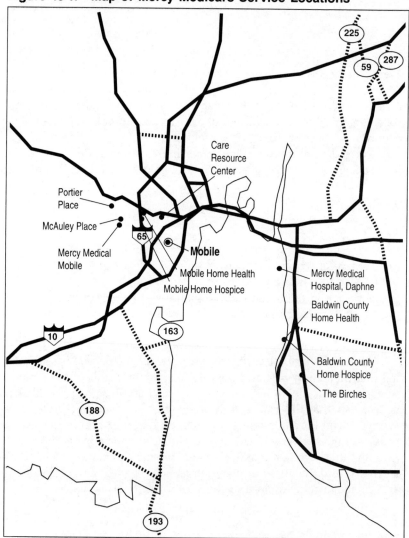

Mercy Medical's Program Areas and Services

By the mid-1970s, Mercy Medical leadership recognized that not all patients needed to be institutionalized and that alternatives needed to be found, and thus initiated a rehabilitation program. In 1982, Mercy Medical approached the State of Alabama to establish a pilot project for a new level of rehabilitation care. Five years later, Mercy Medical was licensed as a 25-bed specialized hospital devoted to medical rehabilitation. Again, in response to another community need, a hospice program was established in 1979 that includes both inpatient and home care components. Then, as an outgrowth of hospice, a home health program was developed in the early 1980s. And finally, in the late 1980s, Mercy Medical entered the field of residential care by purchasing a 60-unit assisted-living facility. Currently, the four main programs are defined as: medical rehabilitation, hospice, long-term medical intervention, and residential. These programs are delivered on an inpatient, outpatient, home care, and residential basis.

Medical Rehabilitation Programs

Mercy Medical's rehabilitation programs include acute medical rehabilitation, progressive care, outpatient therapies, and home care. The Medical Rehabilitation Hospital focuses on aggressive medical intervention and therapy following a catastrophic injury or illness. The term *aggressive* is used because patients participate in rehab therapies, such as physical, occupational, speech, respiratory, and recreational therapy, 7 days a week, up to 6 to 8 hours per day. Because patients admitted to the Progressive Care Unit of the rehab program have more complicated conditions, initially, they may not be able to participate in the aggressive therapies in which a rehab hospital patient is able to participate.

The Hospice Program

Mercy Medical Hospice is the only integrated home care and inpatient hospice in the area under the direction of a single interdisciplinary team. A second 20-bed inpatient hospice opened in Mobile in January 1994 to serve patients in that community. Although the usual admitting diagnosis is cancer, patients with AIDS and other end-stage diseases also are admitted.

The Long-Term Medical Intervention Program

In the Long-Term Medical Intervention (LTMI) program, efforts are under way to identify and focus on subspecialties such as a program for patients with Alzheimer's and other dementias. Other subspecialties will be identified and implemented in the future. Besides patients needing medical intervention on a long-term basis, patients are admitted for both respite and transitional stays.

The Residential Program

In the area of residential care, a 60-unit assisted-living facility known as The Birches is operated in Fairhope, in Baldwin County. A second 60-unit facility called McAuley Place opened in Mobile County in January 1994. Portier Place, a 32-unit independent living residence, opened in Mobile in September 1994. All residential services are tied programmatically and structurally to Mercy Medical's continuum of care.

Mercy Medical also has established a care resource center at a senior citizens center in Mobile. Staff assist senior adults to locate resources through information and referral. In addition, the center provides an adult day health care program and dietary services management. A community care and wellness program provides geriatric assessment and case management either in clients' homes or at the center.

Mercy Medical's Marketing Efforts

Marketing of Mercy Medical to the various publics has been a challenge. In general, most individuals, both medical professionals and the general public, are unfamiliar with the concept of a continuum and how it works. In addition, those individuals who have had some contact with Mercy Medical tend to identify only with a particular program or service. Thus, there has been an ongoing effort to educate various groups about what the continuum encompasses and how it can function to their benefit. Some brochures and literature have been designed mainly to be used with medical professionals; others have been created for the general public. A continuum graphic was developed and is used by speakers and in published materials to illustrate the components of the Mercy Medical continuum and their interaction. (See figure 15-2.)

Daily Operations and Integrating Mechanisms

The four programs mentioned above are the cornerstones of Mercy Medical's continuum. Their integration has evolved in a manner similar to their development and is an area of continual challenges. Informal communication enhanced integration within each service area and among program areas when the organization was smaller; however, as Mercy

Figure 15-2. Continuum of Care at Mercy Medical

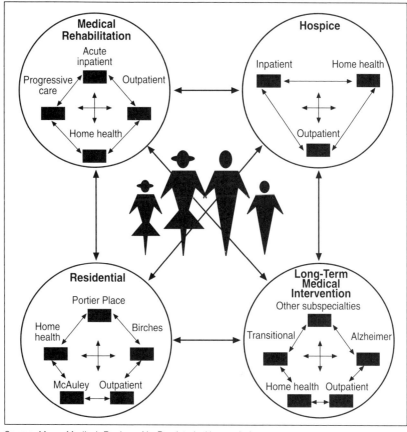

Source: Mercy Medical, Daphne, AL. Reprinted with permission.

Medical has grown in numbers of staff members and locations and in the complexity of its programs, reorganization was required in order for the continuum to operate efficiently and meet the needs of those served. Currently, each of the four programs has an Interdisciplinary Treatment Team. The teams meet weekly and are the primary vehicle for the exchange of information and decision making, with social workers in each area playing key roles in managing care planning.

Patient Flow

An individual can enter the continuum at any point and move from one area of specialization to another as needed, or from one mode of delivery to another. Patients usually are referred to Mercy Medical's clinical programs by physicians or hospital discharge planners. Intake nurse coordinators from the admissions office assess potential patients and coordinate their admission to the most appropriate programs. Admission team meetings are held daily to discuss potential inpatient admissions.

However, an individual can enter the continuum from any setting and move throughout it as his or her needs change. For example, a resident in assisted or independent living may experience an injury, be admitted for rehabilitation, and return to his or her residence receiving ongoing treatment through home health. Mercy Medical staff seek to employ whatever resources are available to meet the needs of a patient or resident, as well as to remove barriers and maximize patient access to services as required. Social workers involved in discharge planning make referrals to appropriate community organizations.

Case Management

Interdisciplinary Treatment Teams are an integral part of the process of case management within Mercy Medical's continuum of care. Each person who enters the continuum is introduced to an interdisciplinary team by the admissions nurse who has assessed the patient/resident and discussed the findings with members of the Admissions Team, which determines appropriate placement within the continuum. Once admitted, the patient is presented to an interdisciplinary team where a process of in-depth evaluation is initiated and a plan of treatment developed. The patient is assessed for psychosocial, physical, spiritual, and functional capabilities by the respective trained professionals on the team. The process is ongoing, and reassessment/reevaluation occurs periodically in order to provide the appropriate level of care on an ongoing basis. Movement of an individual from one of the four programs, or "subcontinuums," to another also is coordinated by the Interdisciplinary Treatment Teams. As long as the patient remains within some phase of the continuum, an interdisciplinary team continues to make recommendations based on the program criteria and the patient's needs.

Staffing

Patient care in all these clinical programs is directed by a physician. Mercy Medical has an overall medical director and additional medical directors for hospice and pulmonary services, along with an organized medical staff. These physicians provide leadership to a staff of health care professionals from a variety of disciplines. Because one component of Mercy Medical is licensed as a hospital, the medical staff is governed by bylaws, and is organized and operates as the medical staff of an acute hospital.

Among the disciplines involved in patient care are: registered nurses, registered physical therapists, registered occupational therapists, registered respiratory therapists, registered speech therapists, registered pharmacists, licensed medical social workers, chaplains, licensed practical nurses, certified nursing assistants, and administrative support staff.

To meet the fluctuating demands of a varying inpatient census, Mercy Medical has adopted a variable budget for nursing services based on hours of patient care per day. The allocation of nursing disciplines to each inpatient program is performed by a staffing supervisor to allow for the movement of nursing personnel resources, as needed, across the various inpatient programs.

Home health staffing also contains a variable component based on a targeted number of visits per day by either a registered nurse or certified nursing assistant. The number of visits differs between rehabilitation and hospice care. Nurse managers are given authority to add to staff as the number of visits per day approaches a given threshold.

Information Systems

Mercy Medical's management information systems (MIS) plans are being driven by the needs of the continuum. To start, MIS is developing a solid, underlying communications network that will link all of Mercy Medical's locations. This communications network will allow for the consistent sharing of clinical, financial, and management information throughout the organization. Hand in hand with this network development is the design of a database that will include protocols for care, as well as outcomes measurements and costs of care.

One goal of the MIS is to improve the quality and continuity of care. It will reduce any confusion or anxiety felt by patients or their families by being referred from one program to another or from one level of care to another. In addition, it will serve to make the continuum function in a more cost-effective manner, eliminating the need for duplicative services and redundant data collection.

Financing/Reimbursement/Budgeting

The area of reimbursement remains a complex and challenging issue for Mercy Medical. Medicare is the primary payer, and four separate provider numbers—hospital, skilled nursing facility (SNF), hospice, and home health—are used. The greatest challenge is in the SNF area, where Mercy Medical continues to be reimbursed at a rate far below its costs. Mercy Medical has had to pursue exception requests with the Health Care Financing Administration (HCFA) to show it provides atypical services, and it has been partially successful in its attempts. It also has sought to diversify its case mix, and as a result, the number of patients admitted with commercial coverage or under a managed care plan has increased. This was pursued on a case-by-case basis until the mid-1990s, and is currently being pursued through contractual arrangements. The LTMI and Residential programs remain primarily private pay.

Managed care does not yet have strong penetration in Alabama. However, in the long term, capitated managed care payment will require that services such as Mercy Medical's be integrated within a system providing a full range of primary, acute, and chronic care services in order to have access to reimbursement under a capitated payment stream. Given the current configuration of the health care delivery system, it is likely that larger acute care organizations will serve initially as the provider locus for allocating capitated payment streams. This has created strong incentives for Mercy Medical to become aligned with appropriate acute care hospital organizations. Its extensive experience and expertise will be an advantage to potential partners in allowing them to bypass a lengthy learning curve and investment process involved in entering into the provision of a new area of service.

Organization and Structure/Administration

Mercy Medical is organized around the four major service areas, with a supportive infrastructure of certain common activities such as financial management, human resources, marketing, planning, development, quality assurance, and others. The organizational structure reflects the clinical areas of specialization and is depicted in figure 15-2.

Relationships with Other Agencies

Another aspect in the development of the continuum is the increasing presence of managed care providers in the local market. Although the development of managed care in south Alabama has been slower than in larger metropolitan areas, the numbers of both providers and individuals participating are increasing. Mercy Medical's continuum has positioned the organization for the future in terms of providing a variety of cost-effective programs that can be used by managed care providers. Mercy Medical currently contracts with other nursing homes to provide hospice to patients in those facilities who have been identified as needing hospice care. Thus, Mercy is developing experience in contracting to provide services. However, the challenge is to develop the integrating mechanisms to allow patients to move from one area of the continuum to another as needed. In addition, communication of the continuum's unique benefits to various provider and payer organizations remains ongoing.

Evaluation and Results

The continued growth of managed care increases the importance of providing integrated regional delivery systems. Strategic alliances and regional systems are compelling approaches to meet the needs of those requiring health care, particularly complex and chronic care, as well as those who pay for these services. Mercy Medical is taking a proactive approach by identifying community needs and the potential partners that, together, may best meet those needs. Networking is not viewed as an end but, rather, a means of achieving Mercy Medical's vision and strategy, as well as preparing for the major changes in health care delivery that are on the horizon. As Mercy Medical has attempted to envision its future, it has determined that as an entity it must establish these vital linkages to complete and enhance its continuum of care.

In summary, Mercy Medical has a unique continuum of programs and services in south Alabama, and is well-positioned for the future. However, achieving the necessary changes in a time of uncertainty within health care in general is always risky, particularly for a small operation.

Patient Example

Mrs. B, a widow, lived alone in Mobile. At age 69, she was still a very independent lady who actively volunteered at the local Red Cross chapter and participated in a number of community and church-related activities. One morning, as she was walking her dog, she fell coming into her yard. After twice getting up and falling again, she called to her neighbors for help. Two of her neighbors drove her to a nearby acute care hospital, where it was discovered that Mrs. B had suffered an acute CVA with right hemiplegia.

After an 8-day stay at the acute care facility, Mrs. B was transferred to Mercy Medical's Rehabilitation Hospital. An interdisciplinary team developed an individualized plan of care for her, and an aggressive rehabilitation program was pursued under the direction of her attending physician. Rehabilitation nursing interventions and physical, occupational, speech, and recreation therapies were provided daily. Dietary services, pharmacy, social work services, and pastoral care also were involved during her stay.

At the end of 64 days, it was determined that Mrs. B would not be able to return home and live independently. She was transferred to Mercy Medical's LTMI program. Determined to regain a greater degree of independence, Mrs. B continued to make progress. She continued speech therapy and her speech improved steadily. Staff assisted her with an exercise program developed by physical therapy staff so that she was able to accomplish independent transfer to and from her wheelchair. One staff member took a particular interest in Mrs. B, working with her personally and encouraging her progress. When the staff member told her that Mercy Medical was constructing a new assisted-living facility in Mobile, close to her former home, Mrs. B suddenly had a new goal.

Five months after her accident, Mrs. B was discharged from LTMI and moved into McAuley Place as one of its first residents. Using her motorized wheelchair, she is able to move freely around the facility, attend the church she previously attended, and take part in outside activities. Her latest goal is to walk with a walker. Not ready to move around the halls, she practices in her studio apartment. In addition, she has become the unofficial hostess of McAuley Place and is very involved in activities. No longer depressed, she has taken charge of her life and is enjoying it once again.

Chapter 16

Fairview

Jeanne Lally

Fairview Hospital and Healthcare Services (now known simply as Fairview) celebrated its 90th birthday in 1996. Under the sponsorship of the Lutheran Church, Fairview began as a single hospital created to serve the needs of disadvantaged Norwegian immigrants in Minneapolis. From those beginnings, the Fairview organization has grown to become one of the largest and most comprehensive health care systems in Minnesota, and successfully operates in one of the most advanced managed care marketplaces in the country. (See figure 16-1 for a map of its service locations.)

With the completion of the merger currently in process with the University of Minnesota Hospital and Clinic, Fairview's annual revenue will reach $1 billion and its service array will cover the entire range of health care services, from home-based personal care and supportive services through the most high-tech quaternary services including bone marrow and solid organ transplants. Fairview remains a mission-driven, not-for-profit organization. Its deliberate and analytic nature is a cultural hallmark, as is its collegial and collaborative management style. It has enjoyed the benefits of visionary leadership throughout its existence, and has been able to attract and retain dedicated and talented management and service staff throughout the organization. Additionally, Fairview has benefited by its strong community and church support.

The organization's recent journey toward growth and integration can be divided into four distinct, but overlapping phases:

- Optimizing the hospital (prior to 1990)
- Reorienting and committing to a health system vision (1990–93)
- Assembling the necessary health system components (1991–present)

Jeanne Lally is vice president of continuum services at Fairview Health System in Minneapolis.

Figure 16-1.   Map of Fairview's Service Locations

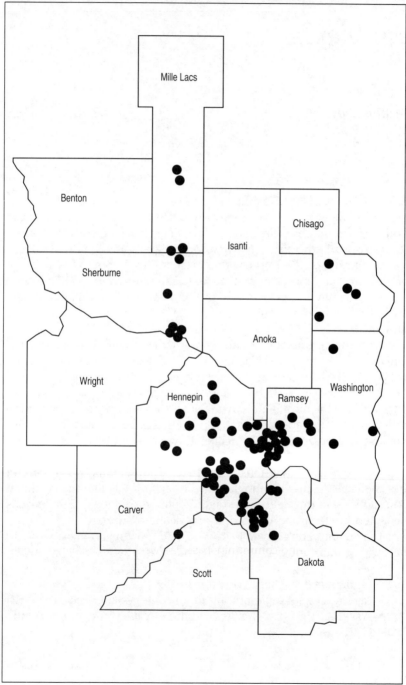

- Optimizing health system performance to meet customer needs (1993 forward)

Optimizing the Hospital (Prior to 1990)

When building and establishing Fairview Southdale Hospital as a satellite hospital in 1965, Fairview became the first hospital system in the country. It was organized and operated as a hospital holding company having up to six community-based hospitals in different regions. Financial margins were primarily driven by inpatient services.

Organizational and operational characteristics of the organization at that time were:

- Each Fairview hospital was a separate star in the constellation, with its own array of services and strategic plan. Some hospitals had overlapping service areas, which resulted in competitive services.
- Corporate services were "lean and mean." The only truly centralized services were financial (accounting, risk management, cash management, and investments). Corporate staff provided consulting or supportive services in other areas to hospital management.
- There was no system identity in the marketplace. Rather, hospital identity was primary and well imbedded into the different communities.
- Hospital services were developed with a revenue orientation. Each hospital was a separate revenue center, and management incentives revolved around individual hospital performance.
- Physicians were seen as customers of Fairview and as potential referrers for hospital services.
- Supportive and/or community-based services were developed with the aim of making the hospital the most attractive hospital in the market (outreach education, transportation services). These services had separate Fairview identities and often "bumped into" one another in the community. This also resulted in inconsistent service availability across the overall Fairview service area.
- The home- and community-based services were discharge-oriented (home care was an example) rather than health maintenance- or prevention-oriented.
- All services were episodic in scope—treating episodes of illness. There was no significant management of conditions or care planning across time, place, or profession.
- In addition to its hospital services, Fairview's continuum of care consisted of:
  - Two primary care clinics employing 25 physicians.

- One-half interest in one home care agency in the metro area and one hospital-based home care department in the rural area, with each providing three kinds of service: skilled care (nursing, therapies, social work), extended hours (homemaker, home health aide), and home infusion therapy.
- One retail pharmacy (owned and developed by one of the metro area hospitals).
- Separate senior services programs operated by two of the three metro hospitals, including services such as lifeline, senior transportation, caregiver support, and senior partners care. Some services were unique to one of the hospitals, some were duplicates. The third hospital had no senior-oriented services.
- Two hospice programs, one Medicare certified and one not.
- A set of "boutique" hospital-based ambulatory programs, often duplicating and competing with one another (for example, hand clinics, spine care clinics).
- Several joint venture programs with other hospitals (a network of ambulatory physical therapy clinics or a mobile imaging service).
- One hospital-based skilled nursing facility providing a mix of long-term care services and subacute care.

Reorienting and Committing to a Health System Vision (1990–93)

This was a period of reflection, evaluation, and articulation of a new vision for Fairview, as well as a period of understanding and communication organizationwide. Crafted by executive management and board, the new vision called for Fairview to transition from a hospital holding company to a comprehensive health care system operating company. The new vision changed Fairview's core business from hospital services to primary care and called for more "systemness" in the Fairview system. It required a fundamental change in outlook and practice, moving from a focus on treating individual episodes of illness on a fee-for-service basis to one on population health management in a risk-based financing environment. And it called for a reduced focus on entity (that is, individual hospital) performance in favor of an increased focus on overall system performance and an increased partnership with communities served. In short, it required a fundamental transformation.

Activities and characteristics of Fairview at that time were:

- Significant communication activities at all levels. CEO Richard Norling and other senior executives spent significant time both internally and externally receiving input and refining the new vision and strategic plan, and communicating the rationale and refining expectations.

- Uneven understanding throughout the organization and, in some cases, resistance to the new strategic direction.
- Development and formalization of a values statement through a sys-temwide task force representing all levels of Fairview employees and constituents. The process was broadly inclusive and resulted in defi-nition of values that represented "Fairview at its best." The Fairview values of dignity, integrity, compassion, and service were defined through a consensus process as Fairview began to think of itself as one organization rather than a collection of separate organizations.
- Embracing continuous quality improvement. Fairview's quality transformation began during this period and provided a frame-work, tools, and skills for evaluating and improving processes across the system.
- Management reorganization was undertaken to provide a platform for coalescing hospital-based services planning and management and for nurturing development of primary care, ambulatory care, home- and community-based services, and systemwide health plan contracting.
- Initial community health assessments were conducted, and the Fairview Foundation was revitalized and positioned to more actively partner with the communities served.

Assembling the Necessary Health System Components (1991–Present)

This is a period of rapid growth, both vertically and horizontally. Primary care and physician integration are key activities. The range of services needed was debated and expanded, and geographic expansion occurred as well. The meaning of the new vision continued to be refined and understood as the organization worked to operationalize it. Fairview changed its focus for its capital investment from hospitals to primary care clinics, ambulatory care, and health plan investments. Key leverage points for system performance were identified.

Activities and characteristics of Fairview at this phase are:

- Fairview aggressively expanded its primary care delivery network through both development and acquisition of clinics and employ-ment of physicians and other primary care providers (currently, 150 physicians), and creation and support of Fairview Physician Associates, a 650-member physician–hospital organization (PHO).

- As majority owner of PreferredOne, one of the area's largest preferred provider organizations (PPOs), Fairview increased its investments to assist it in developing risk-bearing capability and creating a community integrated service network (CISN), an HMO-type organization.
- Strategic and tactical planning continued to deepen. An information services strategic plan was formalized and approved, and Fairview employees throughout the system were connected via e-mail and/or voice mail and began to work on common, connected platforms and systems.
- A change began toward system orientation rather than a specific hospital orientation. Fairview also began to consolidate existing services and eliminate the duplication, rationalizing the hospital-based boutique services.
- Home- and community-based services were administratively moved from individual hospital reporting to continuum services. Service territories were expanded to include the broader Fairview service area resulting in more consistent service provision, single Fairview identity, and reduced administrative costs. Service orientation began to change from postacute focus to primary care support.
- Fairview added durable medical equipment and expanded home care's breadth to include assisted living and hospice service, and retail pharmacy services embarked on an aggressive growth and integration strategy.
- An affiliation with Ebenezer Society brought a full complement of long-term care services—3 nursing homes and 13 owned or managed senior housing units, adult day care, and an array of supportive community-based services for seniors. The community-based services were merged into the Fairview continuum, eliminating duplication while expanding the array.
- Fairview established partnerships with community-based, long-term care providers to enhance communications and broaden network capability.
- Fairview established Community Health Councils to work with community partners and other organizations on community-identified health care issues such as prevention of child abuse, elderly services, and prevention of auto accidents.
- Fairview embarked on a merger with the University of Minnesota Hospital and Clinic. This very significant merger will be completed at the end of 1996 and will bring a full range of tertiary and quaternary services as well as a strong education and research focus.

- Geographic expansion into nearby rural areas and suburbia occurred through acquisition of existing hospital and physician organizations. These were organized as regional integrated care systems, blending physicians and hospitals into single organizations based in their local communities. At the end of 1996, Fairview has two such regional care systems and will add two more upon completion of the merger.
- Fairview's continuum in 1996 includes:
  - An employed network of 150 physicians operating in 29 clinic sites
  - A 650-member PHO
  - Six hospitals (with three more being added with the merger)
  - A comprehensive array of long-term care and subacute care services, including 4 nursing homes and 13 senior housing buildings and the widest array of community-based, long-term care
  - Majority interest in the management company of the largest PPO in the state
  - A comprehensive behavioral services program—the market leader
  - Comprehensive home care and hospice services throughout the service area
  - A growing network of retail pharmacies, currently numbering 10
  - A comprehensive, centrally managed network of rehabilitation services ranging from home to ambulatory to inpatient/subacute

Optimizing Health System Performance to Meet Customer Needs (1993 Forward)

In this phase or set of activities, the key goal is optimizing the performance of the overall Fairview system. Customer needs and expectations are primary drivers. A key focus is to match resources to customer needs, using all elements of the system appropriately and delivering the right service at the right time in the right setting. The key goals became operational integration between programs, seamlessness, overall clinical effectiveness, cost management, and customer service. Emphasis is placed on "managing the white spaces" between the boxes on the organizational chart.

Activities and characteristics of Fairview now are:

- The Fairview vision and goals are simplified, clarified, and restated in customer terms. The vision now reads:

  Fairview and its partners are the health care system in which people and their families have the highest confidence to help

them, throughout all stages of life, stay as healthy as possible
and to help them heal at an affordable cost when they are
ill or injured.

The goal statement now reads:

Fairview and its partners will put our customers above all else.
Our goals are to provide health care services which are:
−easy to use
−affordable
−reliable
−responsive
−comprehensive
and which produce good results.

- Learning and research into health system operations continued.
  Fairview participated in the Shortell Health System Integration
  Study and the Quality Improvement Network, and is a charter
  member of the National Chronic Care Consortium. These and
  affiliations with other, similar emerging health system organizations promoted learning, understanding, and opportunities for
  joint problem solving.
- Services are more oriented to cost management and management
  across time, place, and profession rather than to entity revenue
  production. Management incentive plans are targeted to system
  quality, community dividend, and overall financial performance
  rather than entity performance.
- A key orientation is development of ongoing support systems for
  Fairview's growing primary care core in the effort to ensure its development into a high-performance care system (referral management systems, automated medical records, home and community-
  based services support, integrated product design and contracting
  support, and marketing support).
- Management reorganization was again undertaken to create a single point of executive accountability for the operations of the entire
  delivery system; to promote physician integration; to enhance
  financial planning and risk contracting and risk management capability; and to enhance development of key integrative and support services such as information services, human resources,
  quality support services, marketing, and strategic planning. A subsequent reorganization of the delivery system was undertaken to
  create more formal senior management accountability for clinical
  integration, service line management, and integrated functional
  management, as well as entity operations management.

- Physicians are viewed more as partners and play significant roles at the board level and in management of the PHO and the Fairview primary care clinic delivery system, in development and leadership of clinical pathway and other quality efforts, and in service line planning and management. Fairview's executive management team is composed of six individuals, two of whom are physicians.
- A systemwide marketing department and a marketing plan have been developed. A branding strategy is in place to create a single Fairview identity within the community for all services.
- Strategic initiatives are managed by systemwide councils led by senior executives. Examples include the Human Resources Council, the Marketing Council, the Measurement and Reporting Council, the Quality Improvement Council, the Care Council, and the Integrated Products Council.
- An initial "instrument panel" of measurements to assess overall system performance and progress is designed and in place.
- Contracting efforts grew to bundle payment or accept risk/capitation for a more complete care system, as opposed to selling services on a component-by-component basis. Direct contracting on a risk basis for the Fairview Physician Associates and the Fairview integrated care systems is a reality and is growing significantly.
- Tools and systems are in development, and several have been implemented to promote and operationalize the desired integration across the care continuum (clinical pathways, care management programs, central intake for behavioral and home- and community-based services, central scheduling for clinics, creation of flexible work force teams).
- Information systems activities move from creating common platforms to integrating and standardizing information. A common ADT system is in place, an automated medical record is in development, and an "information warehouse" where information from diverse departmental systems can be integrated for decision support is in process.
- Deliberate efforts to understand that customer needs (both primary customer and health plans) are ongoing. Formal market research has been conducted and analyzed.
- Standardization within operations is a goal wherever possible and appropriate. Functional integration teams and integrated management structures manage key functions systemwide such as imaging, nutrition, medications management, laboratory services, medical records, rehabilitation, social work, and nursing.
- Service line teams have been developed to organize the entire care continuum around the needs of specific patient populations such

as cardiac, behavioral, oncology, occupational health, perinatal, and chronic care.

- Care management programs have been developed and implemented in the acute care setting and selected primary care clinics. A chronic disease care management pilot program has been implemented, establishing care coordinator positions in three primary care clinics to assist integration of the medical and nonmedical needs of patients with chronic conditions.
- A systemwide Pharmaceutical and Therapeutics Committee has been established, and a systemwide formulary is being developed. Pharmacy services have been expanded to clinic settings to assist in clinical processes regarding medications management.
- A Fairview care model has been developed through a multidisciplinary, systemwide task force to serve as a touchstone for clinical providers in all disciplines and across all settings.
- A Robert Wood Johnson–funded project to demonstrate a redesigned, integrated care delivery and financing system for nursing home residents is under way.

Fairview's integration journey is complex and evolving. It may never have a true end point but will always provide opportunity for improvement. At all levels, Fairview has dedicated itself to that journey.

Examples of Fairview's Integration Journey

There has been no predetermined path for programmatic integration at Fairview. However, as the organization gains experience, learning is transferred from one effort to another. Following are examples of how that learning has been applied in three service areas: behavioral, rehabilitation, and geriatric.

Behavioral Services

Fairview hospitals had developed a strong, comprehensive array of behavioral services—from inpatient to community-based clinics. All the hospitals had a significant presence in this area, with one being particularly strong. Fairview program managers and physicians initiated behavioral integration in an effort to solidify their overall presence in the behavioral market because it was increasingly a "carve-out" by health plans. Following are the stages in Fairview's behavioral path to integration:

1. Program managers and physician leaders began to meet regularly to determine a course of action. Eventually, they reached agree-

ment that a consolidated management structure and well-distributed, smooth, continuous program offerings with a central intake/triage function were necessary to meet the behavioral market needs, both clinically and financially. They then designed and proposed a consolidated approach to senior management. This stage of the process took 18 to 24 months.

2. With senior management approval, behavioral services were reorganized to report to a single vice president, and management positions were restructured systemwide to support the integration objective. All managers were given the opportunity to apply for the various positions and the structure was filled, cascading out after the vice-president accountability had been determined.

3. Once the management structure was in place, the programs were modified in accordance with the plan, which included expansion of the central intake/triage, redistribution of certain services, consolidation to remove duplication and increase efficiency, and renegotiation of payer contracts to recognize the systemwide approach.

4. In parallel, the vice president worked closely with key psychiatrists to develop a behavioral PHO and provide the platform for integrated contracting between the Fairview programs and the private practices of the key clinicians. Within this framework, standard credentialing processes and standards, contracting power, and formal ties to Fairview Physician Associates were developed, which allowed for contracting on either a "carve-out" or "carve-in" basis. The current organization is the largest provider of behavioral health services to managed care health plans in Minnesota and is capitated for 55,000 lives on a "carve-out" basis and 10,000 on a "carve-in" basis.

Until integration took place, patients and referral sources would have to talk with multiple points within the system to effect an admission to inpatient or ambulatory programs. Historically, admission criteria, service descriptions, charge structures, promotional materials, clinical protocols, and admission procedures all had been developed at each delivery site and were thus all different. Early efforts, postintegration, addressed these variations in practice with a goal of presenting an integrated, consistent product to the market with multiple locations. As a result, patients or referral sources now can seek system services by calling a single phone number staffed by dedicated system-trained staff 24 hours a day, 7 days a week. Admission criteria, charge structures, and clinical protocols and procedures all have been standardized and are promoted under uniform nomenclature. From a customer perspective, Fairview behavioral services now can be identified as an integrated service delivering consistent product lines in diverse geographic locations.

Rehabilitation Services

Fairview had developed a complete (and sometimes competing) array of rehabilitation services including inpatient, acute outpatient, specialty clinic (for example, hand, occupational, spine), subacute, and home-based. Rehabilitation services integration was approached based on a cost-efficiency as well as a marketplace-positioning motivation. In this case, senior management appointed a task force composed of the key managers of rehabilitation services to prepare a plan of operation that addressed standardization, elimination of duplication, and consolidated management. Based on learnings from Fairview's efforts with behavioral services, the task force was given a clear charge in terms of a financial savings target, a formal chair, and facilitation resources. Following are the stages of Fairview's rehabilitation services integration:

1. The task force met over a period of 10 to 12 months to develop a plan that would meet their goals. The plan called for consolidating/closing competitive clinic sites; developing a consolidated management structure that would standardize operational practices, training, and clinical pathways; and centralizing support functions such as scheduling and staffing.
2. After obtaining management approval through a more straightforward process than had been the case previously (as a result of management's having reorganized to provide a smoother platform for cross-system decision making), reorganization was pursued with processes similar to those followed by behavioral services.
3. After a period of reporting directly to the system chief operating officer, rehabilitation services now reports to a senior vice president for one of the metro area hospitals (not the same hospital where behavioral reports). This continues a practice whereby hospital executives assume systemwide accountability for key services as well as operational accountability for their individual entity.

For 18 months, rehabilitation has been operational systemwide and has accomplished a dramatic reduction in duplicative services/sites, has centralized scheduling, has standardized human resources practices such as training and flexible work forces, and is working on standardizing operational processes across similar sites and integrating practice and documentation between sites. Rehabilitation has been most active in inpatient and ambulatory areas, with significant efforts in subacute and home care as well. Long-term care is still a coming attraction.

Geriatric Services

Geriatrics is a long-standing interest within Fairview. The two largest hospitals had developed social work–based senior programs (some duplicative and competing, and some not), and Fairview had a home care agency and a transitional care-oriented skilled nursing facility (SNF). In an effort to craft an approach to serve seniors well and to integrate the delivery approaches of acute and long-term care, Fairview entered into a small, research and development–oriented joint venture project with Ebenezer Society, a comprehensive long-term care organization. Geriatrics integration is still evolving, but the stages of its progress to date are as follows:

1. The Fairview–Ebenezer joint venture, the Geriatric Care Network (GCN), served as the repository of a large amount of learning about services to seniors, particularly as it relates to chronic care delivery. Individuals involved with the joint venture represented Fairview–Ebenezer at the National Chronic Care Consortium where the learning and product development occurred.

2. Within Fairview, a Geriatric Services Council, chaired by the vice president for continuum services, was formed, composed of members representing all areas of Fairview services, including key clinical and administrative staff. It was a vehicle for systemwide learning, market research, and strategic planning for geriatrics.

3. Fairview undertook consolidation of the senior services provided by the two hospitals and moved their administrative reporting relationship from the individual hospitals to continuum services in order to provide economic efficiencies as well as synergies with GCN. Service territories were expanded to include the broader Fairview service area, resulting in more consistent service provision, a single Fairview identity, and reduced administrative costs.

4. Fairview established partnerships with other community-based, long-term care providers to enhance communications and broaden network capability. These efforts served as the base to develop standardized processes and forms for communicating vital clinical and administrative information between hospitals and long-term care. They also created solid working relationships on which a capitated demonstration project for care for nursing home residents was built.

5. After successful experience with the joint venture, Fairview and Ebenezer executives were convinced that closer organizational ties would strengthen both organizations and position the combined organization well in the marketplace. An affiliation with Ebenezer Society brought a full complement of long-term care services. Management of the Fairview subacute SNF was transferred to Ebenezer. As part of the affiliation planning, the Chronic Care Systems Committee was developed and charged with planning care delivery for chronically ill populations and with oversight of the Ebenezer–Fairview affiliation operations plan.

6. A task force composed of senior management and key staff from Fairview, Ebenezer, and Fairview Physician Associates is currently drafting an older-adult strategic plan that will guide operational planning for all the elements of the system that serve seniors.

Part Four

Conclusion

Chapter 17

The Ideal Continuum of Care

Designing a continuum of care is like a strategic planning process made exponentially complex; implementing it is a challenge of persuasion, teamwork, and managing change. To recap, the ideal continuum of care has the following components:

- A broad array of services, including acute care, long-term care, health-related social support and health promotion
- Services provided in a variety of settings
- Four integrating mechanisms to ensure coordination and continuity of care
  - Clinical care coordination
  - Integrated information systems
  - Inter-entity planning and management
  - Comprehensive and flexible financing

A continuum is customer-oriented and emphasizes functional independence and individual responsibility, while building loyalty and trust in the system. The continuum is also systems-oriented, facilitating continuity of care and capitated financing.

The process for establishing the continuum of care mirrors that of strategic planning and business plan formulation:

- Identify potential participants and discuss participation.
- Establish a Continuum of Care Executive Management Committee comprising the presidents or CEOs of each of the potential participants.
- Create and commit to a shared vision.
- Define goals and measurable objectives.
- Inform/educate board and solicit support for the continuum concept and initial feasibility studies and planning.

- Target a subset of patients for initial focus, with expansion over time to all patients/clients.
- Learn as much as possible about characteristics, needs, and service use patterns of the target population.
- Assess service availability, access, and quality.
- Identify essential services and gaps in services and specify service participation criteria.
- Confirm commitment of preferred service partners (referred to as participating entities).
- Evaluate options for filling service gaps, including assessing structural options and financial implications.
- Set up an organizational structure to assume responsibility for planning, implementation, and ongoing management of operational details, such as a Continuum of Care Planning and Management Committee.
- Appoint a single person as Continuum of Care Director, or vice president, and vest in them the authority and responsibility for coordinating the daily operational issues of the participating entities.
- Create short-term task forces and standing committees to handle the initial planning and ongoing management of specific management functions (such as marketing and human resources).
- Articulate policies, principles, and common operating procedures required of the participating entities and reaffirm the commitment of each entity to adhere to these requirements.
- Determine and implement internal changes needed by each individual service to participate in the continuum.
- Determine and implement operating changes needed to achieve coordination among services, both those within a single parent corporation and across corporations.
- Evaluate the status of each of the three remaining basic integrating mechanisms and set up mechanisms to implement, expand, or fine-tune each of the three integrating mechanisms: care coordination, integrated information systems, comprehensive financing.
- Establish mechanisms for coordinating care across services, such as case management and interdisciplinary teams.
- Develop a long-term plan to implement an integrated information system.
- Modify job descriptions, performance review criteria, and other human resource issues to recognize the continuum.
- Learn current constraints in funding of the continuum and implement all means to maximize available funding.
- Prepare for managed care and capitation, including developing financial arrangements with providers that maximize prevention and comprehensive care.

- Lobby for the ability to pool payment for acute, long-term, and preventive services for use at the provider's discretion.
- Develop financial incentive systems that reward all providers participating in the continuum rather than individual services and reward providers for appropriate use of services by consumers (neither too little nor too much).
- Budget for continuum of care activities and re-establish a budgeting process that enables each participating entity to recognize the financial costs and benefits of collaboration.
- Educate physicians, staff, patients, and family about the continuum.
- Market the continuum, internally and externally, to providers, consumers, and payers.
- Implement a multifaceted approach to evaluation and refine the continuum based on the ongoing findings.
- Continue to inform and educate boards and other governing authorities.
- Anticipate and accommodate ongoing evolution of all aspects of the continuum.
- Incorporate the principles of organizational change throughout the continuum: solicit input from all involved, inform, educate, seek feedback, reinforce desired performance, and continue communication.

Conceptually, the continuum of care makes common sense for everyone: a comprehensive set of services, high quality and affordable, that encourages prevention, health promotion, and individual responsibility and includes long-term as well as acute services to meet changing client needs, with transition between services coordinated by the system and a single bill that optimizes the balance between third-party payments from multiple sources and individual responsibility.

As the population ages and more people have multiple and multifaceted chronic conditions, the demand by individual consumers for a continuum of care can be expected to increase. On a parallel track, as managed care sweeps the nation, employers and payers will increasingly seek contracts with well-organized, efficient, and comprehensive systems of care. The health care organizations that wish to survive and succeed in the marketplace and financial situation of the future will find a continuum of care appealing.

If the arguments for a continuum of care are so compelling, why is the approach not more prevalent or further advanced? Several explanations are possible:

- Although consumers are frustrated with the existing system, very few are sophisticated enough to understand and argue for a continuum as defined here. The desired system should meet consumer demand for care, yet foster independence and freedom and, at the same time, build loyalty to the chosen system. The difference between a paternalistic, underfunded, national health system and a market-oriented continuum of care approach needs to be articulated to consumers, and their input and support need to be solicited.

- Lip-service is given by many health care organizations about the continuum, but few organizations really understand what it is. If and when they begin to realize the complexities of immediate implementation, they may shy away from the task, regardless of how much sense it makes for the future.
- Data on the patient care, satisfaction, and financial outcomes of a continuum of care are available, but not plentiful. Conservatives and skeptics can find reasons to procrastinate.
- The best ways to pool all relevant revenue streams and structure financial incentives to optimize care remain undetermined. Financing is moving in the right direction, but remains fragmented.
- Models of complete organizations and prototypes of continuum components, such as an integrated information system, are relatively scarce; forging new ground is always hard, especially when the subject is as complex as the continuum.
- Implementing a continuum requires changes of mind-set and concrete changes in operations—both are challenging. Envisioning and implementing organizational change requires great commitment and patience.
- A long-term perspective is required; full implementation of the continuum requires several years of planning, intensive attention, considerable resource commitment, and fine-tuning over time.

Despite these challenges, I fully believe that the continuum of care is the right approach for the future. It is the way I hope care will be organized when I or someone I know needs it. It is up to each health care organization of today to decide if it will dwell in the security of old but fragmented care patterns and risk extinction, or if it will accept the complex but exciting task of organizing a health care system that makes sense for the future.